THE FURTHER TALES OF A COUNTRY DOCTOR

2ND EDITION

DR. PAUL CARTER

978-1-955575-28-7 - EBook
978-1-955575-29-4 - Paperback

Prepared for publication by:

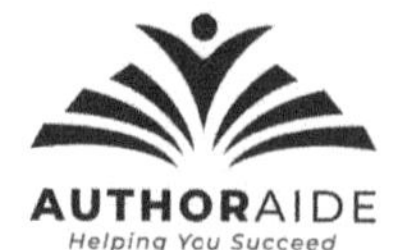

Authoraide Publications, LLC
1603 Capitol Ave, Suite 310 A275 Cheyenne, Wyoming 82001
Office: (307) 459-1803 | Fax: (307) 224-8450
Website: www.authoraide.com

CONTENTS

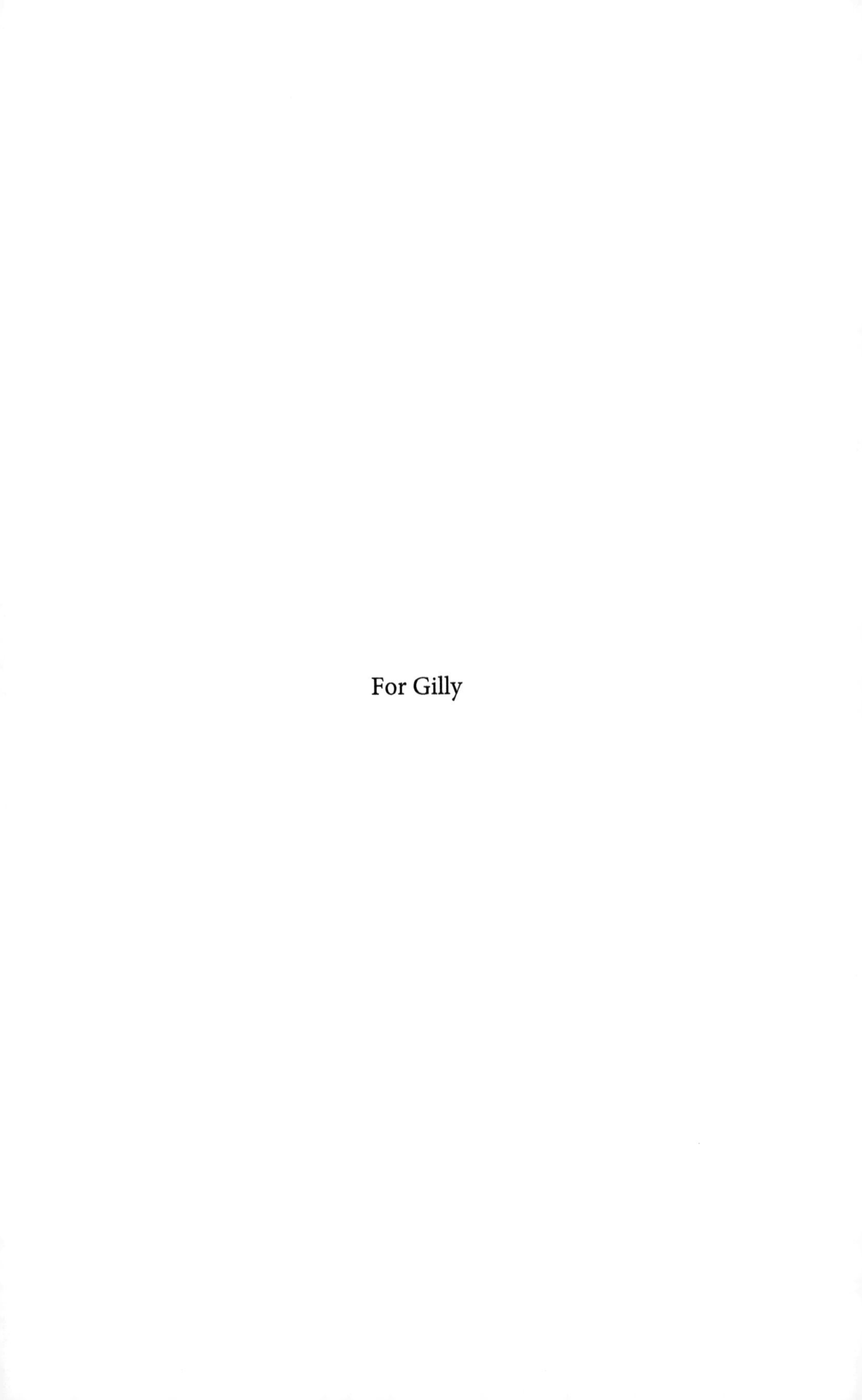

For Gilly

We give thanks for places of refuge and beauty.
Let us find such a place within ourselves.

—*Michael Leunig*
When I Talk to You

ACKNOWLEDGMENTS

I am deeply indebted to all those who have agreed for me to tell their stories. Further, I would like to thank Christina Shennan and Mike Gilmartin for help with my schoolboy French; Richard Day for his one-liners; Clark Stitz for his thoughts on life; Sam Reed and Jenny Darling for their lessons on structure and composition; David Shennan, Tor Roxburgh, and Chris Jackson for their insightful suggestions; Ali-Breeze Jackson King, Julia Stiles, and Angela James for their editing skills; Barbara Thomson for her wonderful encouragement; and Lucila Zentner for the flattering portrait of me.

Last, but by no means least, I also wish to acknowledge Missy Trainor for teaching me everything I will ever need to know about courage.

PROLOGUE

One cold wet night, stuck in traffic on my way to a dinner party, I happened to see a sign on a church noticeboard that said, "Unless you change direction, you will end up where you are going."

Seeing that sign gave me quite a jolt. I was certainly not currently headed in a direction I wanted and decided on the spot to make a change. My marriage had petered out some months before, and I had been going around in aimless circles ever since. I was more than a little lost and had stopped enjoying life.

Over the months that followed seeing the sign, I considered all sorts of possibilities, but none of them really appealed to me. I was beginning to feel I would never find my new direction when, expectedly, the answer was handed to me on a plate by a woman I had been treating for depression in the surgery. She had bounced into my consulting room one day, thanked me for all my help, and then, full of smiles, told me that she wouldn't be needing any of my pills anymore.

When I asked what had led to her miraculous recovery, she said she had finally done what she had been promising herself for years. She had sold her house and was moving to the country.

I was very impressed. She hadn't even moved yet, and already she looked years younger. Right there and then, I silently determined I would follow in her footsteps. I decided that moving to the country would also be the change I had been looking for.

Finding just the right place to move to did not prove to be easy, however. Over many months, I spent every possible weekend traveling the length and breadth of Victoria looking at properties. I saw many lovely places, but none of them sang to me, and I drove a large number of perfectly pleasant real estate agents to distraction with my fussiness about what I was looking for in my new home.

"There must be beauty," I said to them. "And hills and trees, and rolling pastures and running water and a lovely house by a lake in a garden to die for and peace and tranquility and lots and lots of sky."

"You'll be lucky to find all of that," they replied. "Everyone has to compromise eventually."

"But this is my new direction," I would remind them. "Why would I want to compromise?"

Over time, almost all the agents gave up on me, and I was beginning to lose hope of ever finding my ideal country retreat when the last remaining agent took me to see Woongarra, tucked up in the ranges north of Melbourne. On the way there, I wondered whether this would be yet another wasted trip, but I couldn't have been more wrong. There were hills and trees and rolling pastures and running water and a lovely house by a lake in a garden to die for. It was everything I had ever dreamed of, and it sang whole choruses to me. From the moment I stepped foot on the place, I knew that I had found my new home.

As speedily as possible, I sold my house in Melbourne and handed the practice over to my associates. Like the lady who had given me the idea in the first place, I already felt more alive just getting ready for the move. When I eventually drove up the driveway for the first time onto my very own farm, I stopped halfway and danced for joy in the sunshine.

I had always planned on joining a practice in one of the small local towns after giving myself time to settle into my new rural lifestyle. I had imagined that starting in a new practice would take time to organize and require a great deal of negotiation and paperwork, but it didn't happen like that at all. On my very first morning in the country, while picking up some groceries in nearby Dixon's Bridge, I chanced to bump into Felix, the local doctor. He had introduced himself, shaken me by the hand, bid me welcome to the district, and informed me that the job was mine.

"What job?" I had replied.

"Well, the one working with me, of course," he answered with that infectious smile of his. "Oh, and can you be here nice and early in the morning," he added, "because now that you've joined the practice, I wouldn't mind taking a few days off."

As a small child, when people asked what I wanted to be when I grew up, I could never decide between being a farmer or a doctor. Now I am both and can still hardly believe my luck.

And better still, in a small rural area on the opposite side of the world from where I was born, I chanced upon a community of wonderful people who welcomed me as one of their own.

For a little over thirty years now, I have been their family doctor. I have also been their friend, confidante, advocate, priest, batsman, bowler, banker, employer, sounding board, topic of gossip, coach, problem solver, and best man. But the special joy of my relationship with this gentle and loving community is that it has not been a one-way street. While I have carefully looked after them, they have, every bit as carefully, been looking after me.

The following memoirs are about that relationship. They are also about a table and a piano, which somehow became intertwined amongst all the other stories.

While almost everything that follows really did happen, a number of details have been deliberately altered. Names have been changed, timelines jumbled, and personalities altered to maintain and protect privacy or simply at the request of the individuals concerned.

I also freely admit that, among all the reality and mostly for the fun of it, I have also mixed in a little storytelling of my own.

1

ALEX

Alex looked fabulous. She was wearing the bright red crumpled leather jacket she had bought especially for the occasion; her head had been freshly shaved, and she had treated herself to some new ear bolts.

"You look great," I said and gave her a hug.

"You don't scrub up so badly yourself," she replied, looking me up and down. "You know I'd always be yours if you ever whistled under my window."

"Tut, tut," I said, blushing a little. "The things you say, and on your wedding day too!"

Although Alex had given me loads of notice, I was still a little nervous, for I hadn't had much practice at being a best man. Further, in addition to the usual responsibilities of organizing transport, keeping track of rings, and making speeches, she had informed me that it was also my duty to give her away.

I had first met Alex a little over a year before when she opened up the video shop just a few doors down from the surgery. Her family had been residents of Dixon's Bridge for several generations, but she had been living in Melbourne for many years. It was during her absence that I had moved to the country and joined Felix's practice.

The practice in Dixon's Bridge was always busy, and I often felt quite droopy by the end of the day. On these occasions, rather than simply going home to face domestic chores, I would sometimes choose to spend the evening slumped in front of a flick. I loved it when Alex opened up her video shop in the high street shortly after her return to the district, for I could drop in there to pick something up on my way home.

Over time, casual inquiries of Alex about how best to satisfy my evening's recreational needs became passionate debates about the merits of various film classics, which then evolved into sessions with cheese and biscuits with wine on the front counter. To start with, it was just the two of us, but eventually quite a crowd built up until, most evenings, the shop was overflowing.

I guess, however, that it was because Alex spent far more time handing round little squares of cheese and talking about films rather than actually hiring them out that the shop never made any money. As a result, it failed to fulfill its financial obligations and eventually went the way of so many such enterprises before it, which was a pity, for those early evening get-togethers were full of laughter and camaraderie and very much what the doctor ordered at the end of a long and tiring day.

Despite being upset about the closure of her business, together with the consequent loss of her social life, Alex showed good presence of mind. Before the video company representatives arrived to claim back what they saw as theirs, she stacked all the really good movies in the back of her Kombi van and sold off the plain-wrapped ones, which she kept under the front counter for the clientele who like that sort of entertainment.

After the video shop closed its doors, Alex and the van moved in with me. She arrived late one night, long after most law-abiding citizens are safely tucked up in bed, and parked around the end of the old part of the house under the cypress trees.

"Can I park my van at your place for a day or two?" Alex had asked with a fake smile at the surgery a few days before.

"Of course," I'd replied without thinking. "But please, let's first sort out this mess you've got yourself into with your diabetes again."

So Alex and the van moved to Woongarra, and since the back of it was stacked to the roof with videos, she slept in the front seat.

"Wouldn't you prefer a bed?" I asked when the evenings started to cool down a little.

"Is that an invitation?" she replied.

"No, as a matter of fact, it's not," I said, "but come over for a drink," and we sat outside by the lake and had a glass of wine together.

"God, this place is beautiful," Alex said as she looked around. "But don't you ever feel lonely being here on your own?" she asked after a while.

"I don't really have time to think about it," I replied, "what with the practice being so busy and all the farm work. And anyway," I added as I ruffled Hardy's ears, "how could I be lonely when I'm with my best mate?"

Hardy had come into my life some years before when I rescued him from a divorcing couple who were badly neglecting him, and he had become my inseparable companion. When he first arrived, I had imagined making a proper farm dog out of him. In the event, however, I proved to be a hopeless dog disciplinarian. From the very start, he lived in the house with me; and from the very first night, he slept on the end of my bed.

Like me, Alex also fell in love with Hardy. She would fuss over him, and Hardy, being very much a ladies' man, would lap it up. She would stroke his head and say, "How are you going, you great black-and-white poofter?"

"Steady on," he would look up at her adoringly and say. "Being a castrato doesn't mean I'm gay."

Although Alex's occupation of Woongarra was not without its problems, the pluses outweighed the minuses. The mild annoyance of finding that she had commandeered the bathroom and regularly hung her inaptly named "smalls" around the laundry was way more than offset by having an extensive on-site video library from which I could choose at will. I pretended to complain, but in all truth, I liked having her there.

Occasionally, she would come into the house in the evening, and we would have a bite to eat and watch a film together.

"When are you going to move that bloody van off my property?" I said to her one night as the credits of *Kind Hearts and Coronets* rolled up the screen.

"Soon, soon."

"That's what you said a month ago," I replied.

"Yes, well, it's sooner than it was then."

Then one day without warning, both Alex and the van were gone. All that was left to show for her stay were some tire marks in the gravel round the end of the house and a penciled note on the kitchen table anchored down by a bottle of white and a video of *Dr. Strangelove.*

Gone to find love
Ta 4 everything
Luv, Alex

"Well, there you go," I said to Hardy. "I didn't even know she was looking. What do you think of that?"

"I feel a bit sad really," he replied. "She always gave me much more food than you do."

And not only did Alex head off to find love, but almost unbelievably, she found it on the very first evening of her search.

Apparently, when she left Woongarra, she had driven up to the high country with the intention of going farther north the following day. Late in the afternoon, she had chanced upon a pretty camping ground overlooking the headwaters of the Goulburn river and decided to stay there for the night. She made herself a cup of tea and settled back in her old camp chair to watch the sun go down. Below her, in the shallows by the edge of the river, someone was fly-fishing for trout.

"Would you like a cup of tea?" she had shouted down on impulse.

"I certainly would," the answer had come back on the breeze. "And would you like some trout for dinner?"

"Is the pope a Catholic?" she had called out in reply, and the rest, as they say, is history.

Alex and I got into the pickup and headed off for the hall behind the community center where the wedding was to take place. We sat in silence for a few minutes as we drove along, and then jokingly I said, "Shouldn't you be wearing a veil or something?"

"Really?" she said, getting serious all of a sudden. She pulled down the sun visor and began looking at herself in the little mirror. "The scratches don't look that bad, do they?"

"I just meant, aren't brides supposed to wear veils?" I replied.

"Yes, but the scratches aren't *too* bad, are they?" she persisted as she continued to look at herself.

"Barely noticeable," I reassured her. "You look fine."

"Perhaps I should cover them with makeup."

"Well, that would certainly be a first for you." I laughed, and with a scrunch of tires on gravel, we pulled into the car park by the hall. As we came to a standstill, Alex started to pull on a cardigan.

"What on earth are you doing?" I asked. "You'll cook in that thing today."

"I want to cover up my cuts," she replied.

"Cuts, shmutz, who cares?" I said. "Everyone already knows about them. And anyway," I continued, "how many times do I have to tell you that what other people think of you is none of your business?"

"Okay, okay," she said and took the cardigan off again.

"But you could do yourself one favor," I said as she turned to get out of the vehicle. "You could leave that awful old bear in the pickup."

"What?" She turned back to me and hugged the bear tightly. "Leave Spikey?"

"Spikey!" I exclaimed. "He's got less hair than me!"

"Well, he had a lot more once," she said. "And anyway, he has to come," she added. "He's the witness."

There was a crowd of a dozen or so people waiting for us at the entrance to the hall. As we joined them, they stubbed out their cigarettes, and we all went inside.

I had heard a lot about Rhonda in the run up to the wedding, of course, for Alex had talked of little else. Until that day, however, I hadn't actually met the lady in question, and I confess that it was not immediately obvious to me which of Rhonda's particular qualities had stolen Alex's heart away. Perhaps I had just pictured somebody different.

"Hi!" I said as Alex introduced me, and Rhonda crunched my hand.

"Now," Rhonda said to me as she lit a cigarette, "there's to be no fucking about. Just get the rings on, make sure that everyone gets a bit of food and booze inside of them, and then we can all fuck off out of here."

"What about giving Alex away?" I asked.

"Consider it done," she replied.

"Oh, righto," I said as Alex put her arms around Rhonda and gave her a big kiss.

"And no fucking speeches," Rhonda added when she'd disentangled herself. "Now come over here and meet my fucking kids," she added.

So I did. There were four of them, and they all seemed very pleasant young people who were not the slightest bit awkward about being there.

"Your side's a bit thin," I said to Alex as I looked around.

"No, it's not," she replied, "that's my brother over there," and she indicated a fellow sitting at the back of the hall. She waved across to him, and he, almost imperceptibly, nodded back.

Then events unfolded exactly as Rhonda had suggested they might. I produced the rings, Rhonda and Alex gave themselves to one another to the accompaniment of "Wind beneath My Wings," someone put the King on an old CD player, everyone got stuck into the party pies and beer, and then, sometime later, we all fucked off out of there.

After the ceremony and a brief honeymoon staying with Rhonda's children at their various places around Melbourne, the newlyweds went back up to the high country to live. It turned out that Rhonda had a small cabin there, not far from where she liked to fish and very close to where the two of them had first met.

For a while, I lost touch with Alex. Then one evening out of the blue, she phoned up for a chat. At first, I was worried that something was wrong, but she reassured me that everything was just fine.

She called quite often after that, if she had paid her phone bill, and sometimes even drove down to see me in the surgery, if she had enough money for gas. And on the occasions when she visited, I am delighted to say that she invariably came armed with a nice fat trout, carefully wrapped up in newspaper, courtesy of Rhonda.

"Why don't you come up and visit us for a break?" Alex asked on one of her trips down. "We heard about you losing poor Hardy, so a weekend away would do you some good."

"Yes, why don't I?" I replied a little sadly, for unfortunately her information was correct. Hardy had recently, and completely unexpectedly, died; and I felt very lonely without him. I had come home from a Saturday morning surgery to find him collapsed in one of the outbuildings. I had rushed him to the animal hospital, but he had died on the operating table. A ruptured spleen they said, but to this day I still have no idea why.

Shortly before Hardy died, Felix had announced his decision to leave the practice to look after Delphine, his wife, who had fallen ill, so I decided to take the chance of a break away before he finally left. I accepted Alex's invitation and, early the very next Saturday morning, headed up into the hills to see her.

"Get this gear on," Rhonda said to me as soon as I arrived and held out some waders. "We're going fishing."

I had fly-fished in England in years gone by and had really enjoyed it, but nothing had prepared me for the joy of that weekend under the guidance of Rhonda's genius. I spent the entire time thigh deep in cool flowing waters in the company of a master who generously shared with me her knowledge, her skills, and the secrets of her butterfly lightness of touch. I don't remember Rhonda and myself sharing so much as a dozen words that first afternoon. It simply wasn't necessary. We seemed to communicate perfectly without the need for language. By the time we wearily made our way back to the cottage at the end of the day, I felt as if I'd had a prolonged session of massage, relaxation, hypnotherapy, Tai Chi, and mindfulness all rolled into one.

"Thank you, thank you," I murmured appreciatively as we climbed up the slope.

"Don't mention it," Rhonda replied. "Now let's get these fucking fish into a pan, and I'll cook us up a fucking storm."

After the meal, the three of us sat in a circle looking into the dying embers of the campfire. We drank beer and talked of everything from the state of the union to the state of the cosmos. There came a time when Alex wandered away from the fire to get more drinks.

"Isn't she wonderful?" Rhonda said as Alex disappeared into the darkness.

"She sure is," I replied.

"I really admire her," Rhonda continued, "being able to love after what she's been through."

"I've no idea what you're talking about," I said.

"Oh, I'd have thought she would have told…" Rhonda started to say and then stopped without finishing the sentence.

"So do you ever get shat off with being on your own up on the farm?" Rhonda asked, changing the subject as Alex rejoined us.

"Well, yes, since Hardy's died, I do," I replied. "In fact, I'm thinking of getting another dog."

"Dog be buggered," Rhonda replied. "What you need is a woman."

"Been there, done that," I sighed wistfully.

"Well, then it's high time you tried again. There's a heap of difference between someone who sleeps on the end of your bed and someone who sleeps *in* it. I mean, look at me. I was on my own and as miserable as sin for years, and now I've never been happier."

"Thanks," Alex said to Rhonda and put her arms around her.

"I guess you're right," I said as I lay back and looked up at the Milky Way.

"Well, that weekend away sure put a bit of spring in your step," everyone commented on my return.

"It certainly has," I agreed, and over the following months, as far as I was able with Felix now finally gone, I spent as many weekends up on the Goulburn as I could. I already liked Alex, but I also became fond of Rhonda. I valued her shrewd views on life, and I liked her way of getting to the point of anything by cutting straight through all the fucking crap, as she liked to put it.

Then one fateful day, Rhonda went down to fish and simply never came back. She was found, rod in hand, on the banks of the river, and the autopsy showed that she'd had a heart attack. Her death was a shock but, in all truth, no real surprise. She was as wide as she was tall, and she was never without a cigarette in her mouth.

Her final farewell was held near the hut. It was attended by much the same crowd who had been at the wedding. As we took turns sprinkling Rhonda's ashes over the waters of her beloved river, everyone murmured that it was exactly how she would have chosen to go.

For a while, Alex tried living up by the Goulburn on her own, but it didn't work out. After only a few weeks, she loaded up her van and once more headed back down to Woongarra.

I hadn't seen her for a while and was a bit shocked by her appearance. She had lost a lot of weight, and there were many fresh marks on her arms and face.

"And are you looking after yourself properly?" I asked her.

"Of course I am," she said.

"Liar, liar, your pants are on fire," I replied and the next day I got Meaghan, one of the receptionists at the surgery, to organize an appointment for a proper medical checkup.

Over the months that followed, Alex did gradually cheer up a bit. She got herself a purple Mohawk and then, courtesy of the contents of the van, opened up another video shop next to the takeout in Rushby. There was a small flat at the back of the shop, and Alex moved in there.

For a while, the new business did well, and there were even some cheese and biscuit sessions. Alex certainly put a brave enough face on things, but the lines around her eyes made it obvious that she was still struggling with her loss.

Then one morning, Alex opened up for business to find that, during the night, the entire shop front had been spray-painted with "Lezo." It was almost completely cleaned off by lunchtime, but Alex was devastated.

Perhaps it was the distress of the attack, perhaps it was her ongoing financial problems, or perhaps it was simply loneliness that made Alex lose concentration. Whichever it was, just a few weeks after her fellow high-street traders helped scrape the yellow paint off the windows of her shop, Alex crossed a red light on a freeway entrance and went under a semitrailer taking washing machine parts to Sydney.

Looking at the van, it seems impossible to believe that anyone could have survived the accident. Alex did, however, though not by much. Her legs were badly crushed, and she never walked again.

When she eventually came out of hospital, she returned to the shop. The back room was set up by willing hands with furniture that was no longer needed by others and a succession of well-wishers helped with the cooking and the showering. After a while, when Alex had learned to get around in her wheelchair, she even opened up for business again.

I got into the habit of popping into the shop every couple of days or so after work just to check on things. In answer to my inquiries as to how she was going, Alex always said that she was doing just fine, but a sadness had settled over her, and it seemed as if it wasn't just her legs that had been crushed.

One evening she was especially flat, so I decided to cheer her up. "I've been following Rhonda's advice," I said.

"And what was that?" she asked, brightening up a little.

"I've been out on the prowl," I replied. "But I can tell you that between having to run the practice on my own and feeling extremely fussy about who I wish to share my life with, it's been an uphill battle."

"However…?" she cocked her head and asked.

"I *have* met someone," I replied a little smugly. "Her name's Helen."

"That's great. How did you find her?"

"Well, it wasn't actually me who did the finding," I confessed. "An old friend of mine found her for me and passed on her number."

"So come on," Alex said with a faint smile. "What's she like?"

"Everything I've ever hoped for," I replied.

"And have you had her up to the farm yet?" Alex asked with a sideways glance.

"I certainly have," I said.

"And?"

"She came, she dined, she scarpered," I replied.

"Bugger," Alex said.

"*Bugger* doesn't go anywhere near expressing how I feel about it," I said. "But it's early days yet, of course," I added.

"It's still a bugger, though, isn't it?" she said, and I couldn't help but agree with her.

■ ■ ■

Under the pressure of work, I had been fairly socially reclusive for quite some time, but suddenly feeling very isolated after Hardy died, I made a conscious effort to change my ways and became a lot more attentive to my network of friends. I phoned people up and wrote to them. I lunched with them, I remembered their birthdays, and I even held some dinner parties.

And then I found that there are no secrets in a small country community.

"I hear that you're looking for a woman, again," said an old farmer who had been cheated in love many moons before and vowed never to look at a woman again.

"Goodness," I said, startled to find that my affairs were public gossip.

"Well, at the risk of being personal"—he grinned at me through two rows of rotten teeth—"I'd like to ask a question. Are you a slow learner or what?"

■ ■ ■

Over the weeks that followed, I was introduced to lots of lovely ladies. There were many evenings filled with fun and laughter, and there was even, from time to time, you will be glad to hear, an occasional roll in the hay. They were all very pleasant women, but none of them was for me.

"Stop being so fussy," my friends would say. "And anyway, how will you know if you've met the right person when you don't even know what you're looking for?"

"I know what I'm looking for, don't you worry your little heads about that," I would reply. "I'll know her the moment I meet her."

The difficulties in satisfying my exacting standards in the partner stakes gradually had a dampening effect on my career as a social butterfly. Eventually, the local maidens and matrons lost interest in me, the entertainment whirl slowly dried up, and my friends eventually ran out of eligible introductions.

My response was to revert to type. I simply threw myself back into being ridiculously overcommitted with the farm and the practice. Then in the middle of a morning surgery, an old friend from Melbourne had phoned unexpectedly and given me a telephone number.

"This is the one," she said.

"Hhmm…" I had replied.

"The name's Helen, and the rest is up to you," she added brightly.

Over the next few days, I started to dial the number on a number of occasions. Somehow, my fingers always got clumsy, or I found a reason not to complete the connection. Eventually, however, I did have the courage to call, and we organized to have dinner together. So that, just a little over a week later, I found myself driving down to town in heavy traffic through pouring rain to my first and only ever blind date.

"Table for two," I had said brightly to the waiter when I eventually arrived.

"Yes, sir," he had replied with the slightest hint of reprimand. "Your companion has been here for quite some time already," and he then showed me to a table on the balcony where sat the most beautiful woman I have ever seen. I was stunned, and I think my mouth might have fallen open.

"Good evening," said the beautiful woman, and as she smiled across at me, every atom of my DNA swooned.

"For someone who has just met 'the one,' you don't look exactly ecstatic," Alex observed after a short silence.

"Well," I replied after a further pause, "I mean, what if she decides to bugger off?" I said. "I've had it happen before."

"So what do you suggest doing?" Alex asked. "Spending the rest of your life hiding in a cave?"

"Well, no," I replied.

"In which case, just shut the fuck up and take a bloody risk," she said.

■ ■ ■

One evening, I was running later even than usual for my visit to Alex. The carers had already gone home, and I was her only visitor.

"Have you finished for the day?" she asked, and when I said that I had, Alex wheeled herself to the front door and flipped the sign to "Closed." She then reached under the counter, pulled out a bottle of wine, and poured two glasses.

"You shared your story with me," she continued. "So tonight I thought I'd share a story with you. I was married once, you know," she started quietly. "To a bloke, I mean," she added to my astonishment. "It lasted about a year. He was a nice enough fellow, but it just wasn't my cup of tea. I don't know why I started with that bit. I guess I just wanted you to know that you weren't my first best man. Or maybe that was just the easy bit."

Alex took a sip from her glass and looked at the ground between her feet for a long time.

"The story I'm going to tell, though, begins a long time before that. It starts the night of the annual Rushby swimming gala," she said, looking up at me. "I was in the under twelves. I was walking home and feeling really tired as I'd been in quite a few events. A car stopped, and one of my cousins, my mother's favorite, stuck his head out of the window and asked if I'd like a lift home. I knew the mate who was with him, so I got in without thinking. But they didn't drive me home. Instead, they drove me up to the Mullaways. They went up a back road and then down a track into the bush. I screamed and fought, of course, but there was no one there to hear or help. When they'd finished, they ran me home and just left me outside my house."

I sat silently, paralyzed by the story.

"And that's not even the bit that really troubles me," she said with a wry smile.

I indicated with my hands that she was free to continue if she wished. "When I went inside," Alex continued after a pause, "my mother was waiting for me. She asked me what time I thought this was to be coming home and slapped me so hard across the face that she cut my cheek with her ring. 'And look at the mess your clothes are in!' she screamed as she held me by the hair, so I told her what had happened. When I was halfway through, she hit me again."

Alex paused for a while and sipped her wine before continuing.

"She then just kept on hitting me for being such a dirty little slut and for making up such filthy stories about my cousin. And told me that if I ever made up stories like that again, I would really get to know what a thrashing felt like. And then Dad came home, so pissed he could hardly stand and beat the living shit out of her for the millionth time. I ran to my room, got under the bed with Spikey, and never said another word about what had happened. And from time to time, whenever there was no one else around, my cousin would come calling again."

"God almighty!" I said quietly after a long pause. "So how did it all end?" I asked.

"When I was fourteen," she replied, "I decided I couldn't take it anymore, so I just ran away. I stole some money from my dad's wallet, wagged school, caught the bus to Melbourne, and got a job in a bakery. Beverley, one of the ladies there, took me in, and I stayed with her until I was sixteen. She was really kind to me."

"Do you still keep in touch?"

"Sadly, no," Alex replied. "She passed away a couple of years ago. So apart from Mum, there are only three people I've ever told this story to: Beverley, Rhonda, and now you. And since the others are all dead, I guess you're it."

"I guess I am," I said.

"And I've told you because I don't want the story to get lost," she said. "Because then it would just be as if it had never happened. As if it had no meaning."

We sat reflectively in silence for a while.

"So what happened to them?" I eventually asked after we refilled our glasses.

"To the boys, you mean?"

"Yes."

"Nothing. Absolutely nothing. The friend moved away from the district, but my cousin is still around. You know him well."

"Bloody hell! Do I really?" I asked, and she nodded.

"Did you ever make peace with your parents?" I asked after a while.

"I guess I did in my own way, but they never came looking for me, and I never spoke to either one of them ever again. I only moved back when I heard that they'd both died, but I stopped hating them a long time ago."

"How do you cope with this story?" I asked again after another pause.

"By loving and being loved," she replied. "It's the only thing that gets any of us through."

I sat for a while in silence, not knowing what to say. "Well, *I* certainly love you," I eventually said.

Alex looked around the room as if she hadn't heard me. "God, what a mess I've made of my life," she said.

"Isn't it more that life has made a mess of you?" I asked.

"Anyway," she said, "I would like you to take this," and she picked up an envelope from behind the counter and handed it to me.

"What is it?" I asked.

"Just something I've written," she explained, "something I've been meaning to give to you, something I want you to read."

I went to open the envelope, but she stopped me. "No, not now," she said.

"So when?"

"You'll know." She smiled weakly. "You'll know exactly when it's the right time to read it."

"Okay," I said and put the envelope in my pocket.

"And by the way," Alex said as I was leaving a little later, "I love you too."

■ ■ ■

Just ten days later, the district nurse phoned the surgery to say that she couldn't get into the shop to give Alex her morning shower. Sergeant Hogan, who ran the local police station, broke open the side door, and we found Alex lying among all the jumble of the back room and holding her bear.

She had clearly been there for some hours. She was quite stiff, and her cheek was badly mottled from having lain against the arm of the settee. There were insulin syringes and empty pill containers scattered across the floor. Despite that, she looked more at peace than I had ever seen her before, and the lines around her eyes had all melted away. I knelt down by her side and stroked her hair.

"Farewell, dear friend," I whispered.

■ ■ ■

The funeral was a huge affair. Most of Dixon's Bridge and Rushby turned up, and I even caught sight of Rhonda's children among the crowd.

"Where's the bear?" I whispered to the funeral director, for I had expected to see it sitting on the coffin.

"It's inside with her," he whispered back, "as she asked for," and in answer to my surprised look, he told me that Alex had organized everything herself some months before.

The service started with Frank Sinatra singing "My Way" and ended with Anne Murray's "Nobody Loves Me Like You Do." In between, a lot of people stood up in front of a slideshow of Alex in her primary school days and said lovely things about her.

When the slides eventually came to an end, there was silence. I was wondering what was going to happen next when I suddenly realized that this must be the time that Alex had talked about that night in the shop. I stood up and walked to the lectern. I pulled out the envelope that she had given me on that occasion and which, with some inkling of her intentions, I had thought to bring along with me.

I opened the envelope, smoothed out the folded page on the lectern in front of me, and read Alex's message for the first time. It was beautiful, and it was some while before I was able to share it with everyone else.

> My Darling Rhonda
>
> With you by my side, I am beautiful and elegant
>
> Funny and clever
>
> Sensuous and loving
>
> With you by my side, my life is complete

I was about to put the paper back in my pocket when I realized that there was a second sheet, tucked in behind the first:

> And whatever anyone thinks of any of that is absolutely none of my fucking business.

The house seemed especially quiet and dark when I eventually got home that night, so I turned on all the lights, poured myself a whisky, and filled the house with Rigoletto.

"There are definitely times when I really miss that bloody dog of mine," I said to no one in particular.

"Are you alright?" he would have asked me when I got in.

"No, not really," I would have replied. "I've just said goodbye to a good friend of ours."

"Would you like a cuddle?" he would have asked.

"Definitely," I would have answered, and he would have pressed himself up tightly against me, put his beautiful head on my lap, and let me stroke his ridiculous ears.

2

HOO-HOO-HOO

When Helen came into my life, it changed everything. She was all I had ever hoped for. Not only was she beautiful and entertaining company, but right from the start, like Alex with Rhonda, I also felt complete when I was in her company.

A month or so after we'd first met, and completely unexpectedly, Helen created a surprise banquet for me one evening at the farm. It had been a wonderful occasion, but she had then gone home. But now she had agreed to come up to Woongarra again. This time I was keen to impress her with *my* skills, and I was determined to get it right, so I spent a great deal of time and trouble getting ready for the big event.

In a fit of enthusiasm, and ignoring the favorite saying of one of my patients that a tidy home is the sign of a wasted life, I even did some spring-cleaning. To my surprise, I found I quite enjoyed it, but when it came to the detail, I clearly fell below the acceptable standard. Susie, who had looked after the domestic side of my life for the better part of a decade and who had come over to give a hand in getting ready for the big event, was not impressed.

"Stop being picky," I said defensively, "I'm doing my best. There are just some particles of dust that are not visible to the male eye."

I had pictured the evening right from the start. A raging log fire, subdued lighting, candles, sumptuous food, and intoxicating wines. And then, I thought, perhaps I could add a little something on top. Some extra, magical, romantic coup de grâce.

Not long before, I had attended the wedding of the daughter of some friends from town. The ceremony had been held on the lawns of one of the stately homes just south of the Yarra. The weather had been perfect, and at the moment of saying "I do," someone had opened a basket, and a flock of white doves had risen into the late afternoon air and fluttered romantically above the happy couple. It had taken my breath away, and when Helen accepted my invitation to dinner at Woongarra, I was determined that she should dine in a cloud of doves.

To my surprise, the doves were not hard to come by. After only a couple of phone calls, I found myself speaking to William, who, together with his wife, Margaret, whiles away his autumn years breeding miniature ponies out at Mt. Miranda. He also breeds doves and said he was happy for me to pick up a basketful of them around lunchtime on the day of the dinner.

My next thought was of bed linen. To my disappointment, Helen hadn't stayed over after her previous visit, but I was very much hoping that she would do so this time. And if she did, I didn't want to tuck her up in the worn-out, nonmatching, ill-fitting bachelor rubbish that Susie had been trying to get me to throw out for ages. It would have to be something much more suitable for the occasion.

I made the mistake of asking Meaghan and Heather, who between them, look after the reception desk at the clinic, where one should go to get nice bed linen and spent the next few days being "hoo-hoo-hooed" by them.

"I've absolutely no idea what you're going on about," I said. "I'm simply fed up with all my old stuff."

"Hoo-hoo-hoo," they repeated in unison.

Then I did what I should have done in the first place and organized Susie to go and get it all.

"Something really nice," I said to her. "Something classy."

"Not a problem," she replied without hoo-hoo-hooing, but she did tilt her head in a funny way. "And would you like the bed made up with the new stuff as soon as I've got it?"

"No," I said after what I hoped sounded like a casual pause, "put it in the closet. I'll probably just wait and see what comes along."

"Righto," she said.

"Righto to you too," I said back, "and take that silly smirk off your face." Consequently, a few days later, the linen cupboard was filled with brand-new bedding. It all looked really nice, but I nearly fainted when Susie handed me the bill.

"How on earth could a few simple sheets cost this much?" I asked incredulously.

"You said 'classy,'" she replied.

"Yes, but I didn't mean *that* classy," I said, holding the bill at arm's length in the hope that it might look a little smaller.

And with that, Susie wished me well and went off for a well-earned three months' trip to the York peninsula with her husband, whose long service had come due.

Two weeks on my own I could easily have coped with, or even a month, but not three. So I asked Ros at the local store to see if she could find a stand-in. Luckily, her inquiries were immediately successful, and within a day or two, Ros had organized for Janine, a friend of a friend of hers, to come over and meet me. Susie showed her replacement the ropes before leaving, and although I did not know Janine personally, she seemed pleasant enough.

In the days approaching the dinner party, I got seriously down to the detailed planning. In the freezer, there was a large rainbow trout that I had, with great skill, plucked from the upper reaches of a local trout farm, and I was determined to cook it myself.

For once, I decided to dispense with the assistance of Pamela and Carmen, the twins who had so often helped me out with the cooking for dinner parties in the past. I also decided to do without Phill, who usually looked after the serving on those occasions. I love the girls, and I love Phill, but they always upstage me. When they are around, I always feel so useless. They don't set out to do this, of course, it's just the way it happens since they are all so sensational at what they do.

This time I wanted to collect a few chefs' hats for myself.

To be fair, when I told Phill that his services would not be required for the evening, he took the blow well.

"What a relief," he said, smiling bravely and brushing away a theatrical tear. "For I've recently come to the conclusion that dinner parties just do no good for my je ne sais quoi."

The twins, who are both lovely people, or perhaps both the same lovely person, also took rejection gracefully.

"Best of luck," Pamela said. "Don't do anything we wouldn't do," and they both walked away cackling.

In the final couple of days before Helen's visit, I carefully worked my way down the to-do list I had prepared. I rarely ever had time to shop for more than the bare essentials, but I did so on this occasion. To the mild surprise of the local tradespeople, I visited the opportunity shop for candles, the newsagent for napkins, the hardware store for utensils, and the supermarket for vegetables.

Everything seemed to be going smoothly on schedule until, on the night before the big event, I got home to find that Janine had failed to turn up, as promised, and do any cleaning. It was a pity, for the house strongly resembled a pigsty that had been hit by a missile.

Despite the lateness of the hour and feeling dog-tired, I cleaned up the mess myself as best I could. I stuffed all the rubbish out of sight in cupboards, hid things in the spare room, and brought the garden furniture in from outside.

Somehow, I had never gotten around to getting myself a proper dining setting. I had long fancied something made out of recycled timbers, but when I went down to one of the posh inner-city showrooms, with a view to making such a purchase, I found that my mental picture of the cost of a few bits of aged wood glued and dowelled for the purpose of keeping plates and cutlery three feet off the ground was out by a factor of approximately a hundredfold.

The upshot of my visit to the showroom was that I became determined to make my own table out of a tree limb that had fallen across the farm driveway some years before. It had been sawn into planks at the local sawmill and was now stacked and drying in the back of one of the sheds.

The following week I snuck back into the furniture showroom with pencil, paper, and a tape measure. I measured and sketched my favorite table in peace for some time but then made the mistake of also taking some photos. Being before the days of cell phones, I think it was the repeated flashes of my camera that alerted the floor staff to my presence. In just a blink of an eye, or so it seemed, I found myself standing on the footpath outside the store, together with the clear understanding that reentering the establishment would be regarded as a very poor option indeed. Not that I really minded for, hidden safely under the folds of my jumper, I already had what I had gone looking for.

Despite many good intentions, however, I hadn't as yet gotten around to making the table, and in the meantime simply continued to bring the garden setting in from the back patio whenever I had guests.

It had been raining all week, and the furniture was soaking, so I wiped it down and leaned it all at an angle to help it dry off.

The following Saturday morning, the flow of humanity through the surgery seemed relentless. Eventually I got free, however, and tore home to see to the final touches. I even remembered to stop at the bottle shop on the way.

"Have you nothing cold?" I asked.

"Nope. Cooler's on the blink," Jason said. "I heard you were entertaining this evening," he added with a wink as he handed me my purchases.

"Good god," I said. "Is nothing private?"

"Nope," he replied again and gave me my change.

At home, the kitchen became a rare focus of activity. I popped the warm wine in the freezer and started preparing the vegetables. I was quite enjoying getting in touch with my domestic side when the telephone rang.

"When were you thinking of picking up the doves?" William asked. I had completely forgotten about them.

"I'm on my way," I said.

"Well, could you please do me a favor then?" William continued before I could put the phone down. "I've got two hives out in Rusty's orchard. Could you pick them up and bring them back for me? They're all sealed up."

"William, I'm on a very tight schedule today," I said.

"It wouldn't be even two minutes out of your way," he replied.

"Okay, okay," I said and shot out of the door.

Rusty's place, just north of Rushby and near the beginning of the track that leads to William's place, was in fact not the slightest bit out of my way. When I arrived, however, I was asked if I wouldn't mind quickly having a look at the rash on the rear end of the newest addition to the family.

After a brief inspection, I recommended that Sinead's backside be covered with zinc and then went back outside to find that Rusty had put the hives on the back seat of the pickup.

"Shouldn't they go in the tray at the back?" I asked.

"Much easier inside," he replied. "That way you don't have to tie them down."

"Are you sure they'll be okay?" I asked doubtfully.

"Of course. They're all taped up," he reassured me, so I bade him farewell, jumped aboard, and headed off to William's place.

It cannot be more than a few kilometers between the two properties, but the drive demands concentration since the road snakes from side to side as it rises up the divide. Conscious of everything I still had to get ready for my guest, I probably hurried more than wisdom would have dictated. Halfway up Big Hill, I entered a bend a good deal faster than was prudent. Neither I nor the vehicle were ever in the slightest danger, but as the bend tightens up on itself, I did have to adjust the steering sharply. The hives, which until this point had happily complied solely with the laws of gravity and sat solidly on the backseat, now also obeyed the laws of centrifugation, toppled over, split their bindings, and opened up.

I still do not understand why the bees couldn't simply have stayed on the backseat while waiting to get home, but they didn't. Instead, they saw me as a god to be worshipped, and they clustered around me as closely as they could. They covered my hands, they covered my arms, they covered the top of my head, and they covered my face.

To be fair, most of the bees were well behaved, but the pain inflicted by those who were not was unpleasant in the extreme. Fortunately, I have read the *Hitchhiker's Guide to the Galaxy*. On this occasion, it stood me in good stead, for I followed the instructions reputed to be found on the front cover of that publication, didn't panic, and simply kept on driving.

William has since said that when he first saw me, he thought that I was wearing a balaclava. As soon as he realized what had happened, however, he went and put on his veil while I gently turned around in my seat and put the hives back to rights. I then opened one of the windows a fraction, and William filled the car with smoke.

One by one, the bees retreated back to their hives; and twenty minutes later, I was sitting in William's kitchen drinking tea while Margaret scraped the last of the stings from my face.

"Do you think you should call the dinner party off?" she asked.

"No way," I protested. "It would take more than a few insects to get me to change my plans."

"It's just that you look so..." she started to say, but then stopped when William came in.

"I've put the doves on the backseat," he said.

"Well, I hope the basket is properly secured," I replied, and we all laughed. I finished my tea, thanked Margaret for her help, and headed off back to Woongarra. I must have been about halfway there when I caught sight of myself in the rearview mirror. I looked frightful. My face was a swollen blotchy mess, and the one eye that was open was bright red from the smoke.

Gawd, I thought. *All I need is a hump, and I'd get a job as a bell ringer.*

On reaching home, I put any thoughts of my appearance behind me and snapped into action. When I had finished preparing the food, I then went off to sort out the boudoir. So sure was I that the new linen was in the closet that I had reached in to pick it up before I realized that the cupboard was empty. I checked again, but the linen wasn't there the second time either. I then looked in every other cupboard, in every drawer, and even under the bed, but of classy linen I found not so much as a stitch.

"Bugger, bugger, bugger," I seethed at no one in particular as I went outside to find that the firewood I'd ordered hadn't been delivered either.

"Bugger, buggerer, buggerest," I threw my head back at the sky and shouted as I trudged off to the back of the shed to get a barrow load from the stack of green wood that was drying out for next year.

Despite the various setbacks, however, by the time Helen was due to arrive, things were more or less under control. The food was all ready to be cooked, the pigeon basket was hidden behind the settee, Sumi Jo was doing wonderful things with Mozart on the CD player, and the table looked nice even though I couldn't get the candles to light. In fact, when Helen knocked on the front door, I was feeling quite pleased with myself.

"How lovely to see you," I said as I let her in. She looked stunning, and I went to give her a peck on the cheek.

She moved back slightly. "What on earth has happened to your face?"

"Ah, yes, sorry about that," I said. "Bees."

"And the eye?" she continued

"Smoke," I added. "Speaking of which, please come in out of the cold."

"I hope you don't mind," Helen said, "but I've brought along Chanel as well," and she introduced me to a collection of over-excited black pom-poms with a diamante-encrusted collar and a large pink bow on the top of its head.

"Oh," I said hesitantly, "No, of course," and got jumped on.

Underneath Prince Rupert of Hentzau, the stag who graces the wall at the end of my sitting room and smiles down on everyone with the regal expression, *Monarch of the Glen*, on his face, there is a huge fireplace. It is an impressive structure, and some people have even been kind enough to call it baronial. The wide hearth is usually a cheerful place to stand in front of and toast one's legs by the heat of crackling logs. That night, however, there was neither crackling, nor indeed anything cheerful about the logs, which I had brought round from the back of the shed. They simply lay on the bricks and sulked.

"Charming," Helen said as she looked around, "but would you mind opening a door?"

"Yes," I agreed. "It is a bit smoky, isn't it?"

I opened a door to let the smoke out and then helped Helen put her coat back on again against the chill.

"Glass of wine?" I asked.

"That would be lovely," she said.

On opening the freezer, I found that the wine bottles had done what they always do when they are left unattended for several hours at minus twenty.

"Bugger, buggerante, buggerissimo," I hissed to myself in a whisper as I put the fractured bottles in the bin. I stood for a moment paralyzed by indecision and then, in a moment of inspiration, remembered that, while tidying up earlier in the week, I had seen some of Mario's homebrew underneath the bottom shelf in the pantry. A year or so before, Mario, the head of the local Italian dynasty, had given me some of his homemade wine as a present. I hadn't liked it much but hadn't had the heart to throw it away. I quickly unscrewed one of the flagons, filled a decanter, and sauntered back into the sitting room as cool as a cucumber.

Helen took a small sip. "Goodness," she said with the slightest of starts and then set her glass down on the table. "Most unusual," she added.

"I'll go and get the food going," I said.

"Want any help?" she asked.

"No, no," I replied. "Everything's under control."

Within a few minutes, the vegetables were in the oven, and the plates were in the warmer. I felt cautiously proud of myself. I had always imagined, from what others had said, that cooking was trickier than this. I went back through to the sitting room and chatted with Helen.

The roof of my mouth was, once again, getting used to Mario's brew when a thought flashed through my mind. Five seconds later the fish was out of the freezer, ten seconds later it was under the grill, and fifteen seconds later, I was back chatting with Helen and drinking Mario's paint stripper as if nothing had happened.

"Are you sure that there's nothing I can help with?" She smiled.

"No, thanks, I can manage." I smiled, and not long after that, I put a meal in front of each of us.

"Gosh, that looks nice," Helen lied as we sat down, "but before we start," she continued, "would you have a towel I could sit on?"

"Of course," I replied. "I think I'll get one for myself as well."

And almost immediately after we cheerily clinked our glasses together, it became obvious that while the fish was burnt on the top, it was still deeply frozen underneath.

"I love frozen fish," Helen joked and then, with a puzzled look on her face, pulled something out of her mouth.

No one has ever told me, and I have never seen it written down anywhere, that you should remove cling wrap before putting vegetable dishes in the oven. Perhaps it is just seen as a given. Anyway, it simply never occurred to me that it was necessary, so we spent the rest of the meal silently picking small pieces of shriveled plastic from between our teeth.

We had pretty much finished the thawed parts of our fish when Helen sniffed a couple of times and said, "I hope you don't mind me asking, but is there a funny smell in here?"

I lifted my nose to the air and feigned ignorance.

Never having owned doves, it wasn't until I put them on the back seat of the pickup that I realized how much they smell. For months afterward, anyone getting into my pickup would wrinkle their nose and say, "I hope you don't mind me asking, but what in God's name is that awful stink?"

"There *is* a smell, you know," Helen persisted, "and it's coming from behind that couch."

Since that evening, I have come to learn that among Helen's many fine attributes is a sense of smell that would put the average beagle to shame, and that if she ever turns away from teaching, she would have a ready-made second career at the airport sniffing luggage. But I didn't know that then, and although the smell was pretty obvious, even to me, I was about to protest the innocence of my sitting room when I looked at her wrinkled nose and decided instead that the time had arrived for the magical, romantic coup de grâce.

In answer to Helen's comment, I nonchalantly sauntered behind the couch, reached down, and threw open the basket. I then looked up at Helen, spread my arms wide, and said, "Surprise."

A cloud of white doves burst out of the basket and fluttered around Helen's head. They settled on the table close by her and even on her shoulders. She reached out her hands, and I held my breath as birds flew onto both of her palms. Helen was quite overcome with emotion. She looked up at me as tears trickled down her cheeks.

"Oh, Paul, you are wonderful," she murmured.

At least, that was what was supposed to happen, and that was certainly what I had seen in my imagination all week. What actually did happen was nothing.

"Surprise what?" Helen said as I looked down on the backs of eight birds huddled motionless in the bottom of the basket.

"Out, out," I hissed at them and tipped the basket on its side.

"What on earth are you doing back there?" Helen asked as the birds rolled out and stood quietly by my feet.

Helen poked her head over the back of the couch and started to laugh. "What on earth are you doing?" she repeated.

"These are supposed to be flying around your head in an enchanting cloud that makes me irresistible to you. They have been hired specifically for the job and are not going to get away with shirking their duties," I said, and I scooped one up and threw it in the air. After just three flaps, it landed on the back of the couch, got itself comfortable, fluffed up its feathers, and shat on the cushion.

Later, as I cleared away the table, Helen lied again. "That was a wonderful meal," she said and began to cry.

"Please don't be upset," I comforted her.

"I'm not upset," she said. "It's just that the smoke has built up again," so I opened the door once more.

"Could you please get my coat for me?" she asked.

"Are you leaving?" I asked sadly.

"Why on earth would I be leaving?" She laughed. "I'm just cold."

"I am so sorry," I said after a moment or two's pause. "I tried so hard."

"I know, and that's what has made it all so wonderful," she said and reached across the table and touched my hand in a way that sent lightning bolts all round my body.

And then we picked up the birds and stroked them on our laps, drank Mario's wine until it tasted okay, and laughed late into the night until, totally unexpectedly and without any warning, Helen glanced down at her watch and told me that it was time for her to go. I was stunned.

"Oh, no. Please don't," I pleaded. "I would really love you to stay."

"I know, Paul." She looked up at me. "But it has been less than three years since Richard passed away," she continued. "I really thought I would be ready to be with someone else by now, but I can feel that I'm just not there yet. I am so sorry, I really am."

I heard the words "Don't be silly. There's no need to apologize" come out of my mouth.

"Thank you for being so understanding." She smiled back at me as we went outside. We shook hands, and Helen loaded Chanel back into her car. "It has been a really wonderful evening," she said. "We must catch up soon."

"We sure will," I said, with a stiff smile on my face, and I waved at her taillights as they disappeared down the driveway.

"Sod it," I shouted up at the stars as I turned to go in, "and shit!" I swore at the pigeons as I stomped off to a bed, which seemed colder and emptier than I could ever remember. I ached to have Helen there next to me, and I was conscious of her absence all night.

Sometime overnight, the birds remembered how to fly again; and perched high on the sills of the clerestory windows, they were the very devil to catch the next morning. I was also impressed at how thoroughly they had carried out my final communication to them of the night before.

Forgiving them their poor start, and also since William wasn't allowed to have them back as Margaret said he already had too many of them, the birds stayed on at Woongarra. I took them out to the old dovecote in the farmyard where they lived peacefully for many years until one day, literally out of the blue, a local hawk took a fancy to them, and one by one, they disappeared.

■ ■ ■

The day after Helen's visit, and looking for something to do to distract me from the disappointment of the night before, I made a start on the paperwork piled up on my desk and paid off a few outstanding bills. In doing so, I idly flicked through the stubs in my checkbook and realized that one of them was blank. I am normally quite good about that sort of thing, so the following Monday, I contacted the bank to get the details of the mystery check and found out, to my surprise, that it had been cashed for a thousand dollars.

Meaghan did a phone round for me and, in almost no time at all, found that the check had been presented to the local garage.

"Who cashed it?" I asked the garage proprietor on the phone a few minutes later.

"Your stand-in housekeeper," he replied. "Why, is there a problem?"

"No, no, not at all," I reassured him. "Did I remember to sign it by any chance?" I asked.

"Yes, but come to think of it, it wasn't your usual scrawl. Are you sure there isn't a problem?"

"No, no, there's no problem at all," I reassured him again and rang off.

A nicely spoken lady, whose voice had clearly been recorded by the telecommunications company for exactly that reason, regretted to inform me that Janine's number had been disconnected. On my way home, therefore, I called into the local store and asked Ros to pass on a message through the bush telegraph that unless there was a bulky envelope and a pile of bed linen at the practice by the following day, I would be having a quiet word with Sergeant Hogan. Ros was very apologetic about the whole affair, but of course, it was really nothing to do with her.

To my complete surprise, a fat envelope did appear at reception the following morning, having been left there by a friend of a friend of a friend. Of bedding there was none, but an envelope was better than nothing, and I resolved myself to settle for that, if need be.

Then, later that day, Chloe, came in crying and very distressed. She is a lovely girl, who serves behind the counter of the hardware store. She asked for a certificate, sobbing that she was too upset to go to work. When she eventually settled down, I asked what the problem was.

It appeared that she was planning to get engaged to Drew, who works in the timber department, but that they would now have to postpone the festivities as the money they had saved up to pay for the engagement party had gone missing. Apparently, she had put the money in her savings account but now found that it was empty. Chloe said that although it was a terrible thing to say, she suspected her mother, who had done something like this before to another family member.

"And how much money are we talking about?" I asked.

"A thousand dollars." Chloe sobbed.

"And when did this happen?"

"This morning." She snuffled through a tissue.

"Ah," I said and then asked after a pause, "and your mother's name would be…?" and got exactly the answer I was expecting.

"Mmm," I murmured pensively. I sat for a moment with my head bowed. For just a brief, fleeting moment, I thought of feigning ignorance, but then sadly opened the top drawer of my desk and took out the envelope.

"In which case," I continued reluctantly as I handed it over, "this probably belongs to you."

▪ ▪ ▪

"So how did it go?" Heather eagerly asked a day or so later when she returned from a break. She then looked at me and added, "And what in God's name have you done to your face?"

"Bees," I said. "It's much better now."

"Really?" she said, peering at me from all angles, "but anyway, how did it go?"

"How did what go?" I replied nonchalantly.

"Don't be a daft pillock," she said. "You know what I mean. How did *it* go?"

"*It* didn't, in any sense, go at all," I said with a sigh. "If you really want to know, it was a complete disaster. Why I tried to do it all without Phill and the twins, I shall never know. Helen spent the entire evening sitting on a wet seat being served inedible food and undrinkable wine by a man she could hardly recognize in a cold, smoke-filled room whilst picking bits of plastic out of her teeth in the company of birds that had forgotten how to fly."

"Brilliant!" Heather laughed. "Absolutely brilliant."

"What on earth's so brilliant about that?" I asked in amazement.

"Well, how could she not fall in love with someone as completely useless as that?" She laughed and then gave me a big hug and went back to reception.

RECIPES FOR DISASTER

Truit avec Colombe

1 trout
1 lemon
1 packet sliced almonds
¼ tub garlic butter
Vegetables
1 basket doves

1. Defrost trout if frozen.
2. Fill with almonds and lemon slices. Smear with butter.
3. Wrap in foil and place in oven.
4. Remove Glad wrap from vegetables before cooking.
5. Allow doves time to warm up.

3

TAMAS

Eduard was a likeable man who had a dental practice in Melbourne. I didn't see him very often, but occasionally, he would visit the surgery when he was spending time at his property just outside Stoney Creek.

He came in one Saturday morning and asked me for a favor.

"I wonder if you would be prepared to be involved in the care of my dad?" he said. "His usual GP's down in town, but he and my mom spend almost all their time up here now. He's getting very frail, and I feel he should have someone looking after him at this end too."

"Yes, of course," I replied. "I'll get one of the girls to give him a call and make an appointment."

"I was hoping you might visit him at home," Eduard said, and I replied that I'd be happy to do that too.

A home visit was duly organized, and when I called there early the following week, Tamas—dental surgeon, raconteur, inventor, bon vivant, and daffodil grower—came into my life as a breath of fresh air.

Tamas had known of the lymphoma for many years, but for most of that time, it had hardly troubled him at all. Recently, however, for reasons not clear to the medical profession, it had exploded into life like an erupting volcano and scattered bits of itself all over his insides. Within just a few months, he had been forced to cut down dramatically on his Melbourne practice and now lived in semiretirement on his hobby farm next to Eduard's place.

I got into the habit of popping in to see Tamas on a regular basis. The property was awkwardly out of my usual round, but if I got the timing right and arrived around lunchtime, I was always assured of a large plateful of something warm and filling made by Lujza. I always made a point of complimenting my hostess on her cooking, and at the end of each visit, Tamas's wife would then insist that I take away enough food for my evening meal as well.

I once took a risotto dish of my own creation with me on my visit in an attempt to balance up the hospitality. I felt really annoyed with myself over the complete mess I'd made of things the night Helen came up to the farm for dinner and was determined to improve my cooking skills in the hope that she might have the courage to come again.

I began by borrowing some cookery books from Meaghan and Heather. Unfortunately, the books were useless to me as they assumed that I already knew how to do everything and what everything was called. I then sought the help of various friends and asked each of them to provide me with a recipe that they thought *I* would be able to cope with.

"Imagine," I said to them, "that I have very little kitchen equipment—"

"Well, we know that," they interrupted.

"And no cooking skills whatsoever—"

"Well, we know that as well," they interrupted again.

"And very little time to prepare—"

"You mean you're actually going to try some cooking?" They sniggered.

"I don't see what's so funny about that," I replied defensively, but they just chuckled in reply.

Despite the mirth, however, my friends did come through. They stuck rigidly to the brief they had each been given and produced old family favorites that they thought even I would be able to manage. Over time, I collected quite a number of them. *Recipes for disaster*, I called them, and I kept them in a folder in the kitchen.

No one presented me with a recipe for eggs and bacon or corn on the cob, but as was explained to me, some things have no recipe, you just do them.

This risotto was one of those recipes, but I'm not sure it was quite the success I was hoping for because although Lujza and Tamas said "thanks," they also said that I needn't go to any more trouble on their behalf in the future.

Although the reason for my calling out to the daffodil farm was Tamas's ever deteriorating health, I very much looked forward to the visits. Not only did I like Tamas and Lujza right from the start, but after Tamas and I had completed the medical part of my visit, and while Lujza was putting the finishing touches to lunch, Tamas would take me outside to show me the latest project he was putting together in his workshop. That workshop was a wonderful place, and in it Tamas must have had every piece of metalworking equipment that has ever been invented. He proudly said that he could cut, fold, twist, shape, and bend steel into whatever shape took his fancy.

"Where on earth did you learn how to do all this?" I asked in admiration as I inspected the newly completed roller track that he'd invented for getting heavy shopping from the boot of the car to the back door.

"What do you mean?" he answered. "It's just big dentistry. I look to see what the problem is and then work out how best to fix it. Come on over one evening, and I'll show you how to do it if you like."

"I would like that very much," I replied and, over the following months, spent several wonderful evenings under Tamas's tutelage, making steel sculptures for my garden.

"They're fabulous," I said on the day of their unveiling.

"And as you see," he said as he looked around with a smile, "they have filled up some of the gaps in your garden."

Tamas and Lujza were charming and cultured people, and they lived in a house completely lined with books. They loved talking about literature and music, and they conversed between themselves in whichever of half a dozen languages seemed to best suit the topic. I enjoyed their company enormously, discussing and arguing about everything under the sun, and often had to get a move on to make my afternoon surgery in time.

Although I always went to their house to see Tamas, Lujza, who I also acquired as a patient, came to see me at the surgery. While I loved her dearly, my heart sank whenever I saw her name on the appointment list. She always took so long and invariably put me way behind schedule.

Whatever the season, she wore an ankle-length overcoat and headscarf. Whatever the time of day, she carried at least three large bags in either hand. She reminded me of every picture I have ever seen of a refugee fleeing from somewhere to somewhere else and taking all their worldly possessions with them.

"And how's my favorite bag lady?" I would say.

"Well, just wait and see what I have brought for you today," she would reply, and then produce prosciutto and jars of homemade pickled mushrooms and impossibly sweet biscuits, and long ago–recorded Hungarian operas, and once, some gloves she had knitted especially for me.

"I always think of you." She would smile as she spread her fare across my desk.

"I can see that," I would reply, and then we would jointly begin the exhaustingly slow process of removing her outer layers so that I could examine her and start addressing the neatly written list of problems and complaints she had always carefully prepared for me.

When we eventually got to the bottom of the list, I would then help her back into her garments, thank her for her gifts, and start steering her gently toward the door, hoping she wouldn't remember anything else that needed my attention.

"You are like a son to me," she would say at the door and give me a peck on the cheek before she went.

■ ■ ■

In Hungary, at the time when Tamas qualified, all a dentist had to do to establish a practice was simply hang up a brass nameplate and roll up his shirtsleeves. Tamas chose to set up his rooms in one of the inner-city areas of Budapest, not far from the riverbank. Through hard work, skill, and the support of his young bride, the practice thrived. Although the area of the town where the practice was located was not particularly well to do, word of Tamas's skill spread rapidly; and within a few years, he had more work than he could handle.

It was right at the point of him feeling comfortably established, with a young family and a successful practice, when everything came to a grinding halt. At first, Tamas somehow imagined that the political upheaval engulfing his country might blow over without affecting either him or his family. When Russian tanks rumbled over the border and headed for his city, however, he realized that his original assessment had been wildly off the mark.

Recognizing that there would be, at best, only a small window of opportunity of escaping Russian occupation, Tamas acted with speed. The very same day that the invaders crossed the border, he packed as much of his equipment as he could into the boot of his Citroen, strapped his dental chair on to the roof rack, loaded up Lujza and the boys, and headed out of Budapest as fast as possible.

The journey to the west was slow going, thanks to all the other fleeing traffic, but Tamas was rewarded for his quick thinking by crossing the Austrian border just an hour or two before it was closed.

I understand that the rest of the journey to Vienna, where they had arranged to stay with relatives, was for Tamas and Lujza a roller-coaster ride of elation at having escaped and of sadness at having to leave.

Tamas's new practice in Vienna was every bit as successful as its predecessor. After a couple of years, however, when it became clear that there was going to be no quick way back to their mother country, Tamas and Lujza decided to get right away from Europe and give the boys a completely new start. This time, however, rather than pack everything up again, they simply sold the practice, bought four tickets, got on a boat, and headed down under.

The move to Australia proved to be a happy one, and Tamas avoided the two-year bond by having paid for his family's passage. Lujza liked her new house in Fitzroy, the boys settled into their new school, and the new Australian practice, which Tamas set up as soon as they arrived, proved to be his busiest yet. With Lujza at the reception desk and Tamas in the surgery, they drew, from miles around, all their compatriots who had also managed to escape.

Lujza and Tamas loved Australia and took out citizenship as soon as they could. They became experts on cricket and footy and would happily bore the pants off anyone by talking about their newly appointed heroes. Not everything worked out perfectly, though. Just a few years after they arrived, Tamas Junior fell ill with meningitis and sadly never recovered.

When Eduard, the younger son, went off to dental school, the house in Fitzroy seemed very empty, and Lujza and Tamas reasoned it was time for a change. They decided to keep the place in town, but they also bought the farm at Stoney Creek to which they would escape at weekends.

Although the practice in Fitzroy was always frantically busy, Tamas stayed as fiercely independent as he had before and continued to work single-handedly right up until the time when the newly qualified Eduard joined the practice. It was a match made in heaven, and Tamas and Eduard, who had always got on well, worked happily together for many years without so much as a cross word.

"I think I'll have to completely retire soon," Tamas sadly said to me on one of my visits, as he lay on his bed looking down at his swollen and bruised legs and tummy.

"Don't you think it's ridiculous that he hasn't already done so?" Lujza looked at me and asked. I agreed, and eventually, and extremely reluctantly, Tamas handed over the reins of the practice to his son.

"Talking of handing over to the next generation," Tamas said with a twinkle in his eye, "I hear that there's going to be a new dentist in Dixon's Bridge."

"There certainly is." I smiled at him, for by strange coincidence, at about the time I started visiting Tamas, and before I met Helen, another dentist had come into my life. Completely unexpectedly, I'd been approached by a surprisingly young lady dentist who had recently moved into the area. She had asked if she could rent Felix's old consulting room and kit it out for use as a dental surgery until I found someone to fill Felix's shoes. She was vivacious, curvaceous, pretty, and I'd immediately said "yes."

"I hear she's very 'ooh la la,'" Lujza said with a wink. "You're on your own. Perhaps you should have her over for a meal one night."

"She's certainly very pretty." I laughed. "But no thanks. Anyway, I recently had a really lovely lady over for dinner and made a complete disaster of it."

"Worse than the risotto, I think it was, you brought here once?" Tamas asked.

"Much, much worse," I replied.

"Goodness," they both said. "We didn't realize that was possible."

▪ ▪ ▪

Under Ooh la la's guidance, Felix's old room was duly converted to suit its new use, complete with all the necessary equipment and fittings. The room was painted in three fetching shades of purple, and the finished article looked very professional indeed with all the certificates hung up across the back wall.

We came to the arrangement that, in the first instance, Heather and Meaghan would keep track of the dental appointments, as well as my own, and also handle the money side of things for her. The new dentist insisted, in view of the cost of the setup, that, at least to start with, patients should pay up in full before she saw them.

The announcement of the arrival of a new dentist in town caused a great deal of excitement, and even before the grand "open wide please" day, as it was called locally, she was booked out for weeks ahead.

"I understand that the launch of the new dental service was not without its problems," Tamas said with just the hint of a smile when I visited him some days after the event, and he was spot-on.

Despite all the buildup, the start of the new dental service proved to be a considerable disappointment for two reasons. The first was that the new dentist failed to put in an appearance, and together with all the money that we had collected on her behalf, has never been seen again. The second was that, on the very same day, I received all the bills for the fit-out of the room.

Unlike Ooh la la, however, Tamas was keen to keep working and asked that an exception to his retirement from his city practice be made for any patients who chose to travel to Stoney Creek to see him. Thinking that no one would come, Lujza and Eduard were only too happy to agree, but they were wrong. Initially, it was just the occasional patient who made the pilgrimage to the country. But as the weeks went by, the number of visitors grew into a regular flow, and eventually the storage area at the end of the veranda had to be converted into a makeshift waiting room.

"This is ridiculous," Lujza would say again.

"This is wonderful," Tamas would reply, and even as his illness progressed, he continued to work.

"Can't you stop him?" Lujza asked.

"I don't think I can," I replied.

Little by little, however, the lymphoma started winning. Tamas became ever more breathless, and his legs and tummy grew increasingly swollen and bruised. Then one morning, without any need for argument, Tamas's career came to an end. Having bled into his eyes during the night, he woke up barely able to see.

With no patients to worry about, Tamas went into a decline.

"What's the point in being alive if I can't help others?" he would say. "Perhaps this is the time for you to care for yourself," we would all reply. "I don't think I know how to do that," he would say.

"Well, now's the time to practice," we would reply again.

And then, just a month later, Tamas went peacefully to sleep one night and simply never woke up.

A couple of days before he died, on one of my regular visits, he beckoned me over to sit on the edge of his bed. "I imagine that many people must look back on their lives at this point and say to themselves, 'What was that all about?'" he said, "or even 'Thank the Lord that's over,' but not me."

"Why, what do you say?" I asked.

"I say, 'Now that was bloody good fun,'" he said quietly and held my hand.

The funeral, held a few days later at the cathedral, was a huge event. It seemed as if every Hungarian in Melbourne wanted to bid Tamas farewell. The service comprised eulogy after eulogy of praise for both the man and his services to his community. Then when all the words had been said, Tamas departed on his last journey, drawn, as he had always said that he wanted to be, by four black horses with plumes on their heads.

Not long after the funeral, in a lovely gesture, the Hungarian community commemorated Tamas's life and work with a plaque in the rose garden in the park across the road from the practice. Eduard was so moved by it that he felt he'd like to see his father's life's work honored by his fellow professionals also.

"Wouldn't it be nice if the dental community also recognized Dad's contribution?" he said as he stood with his mother at the unveiling.

"I don't think that's a good idea at all," his mother unexpectedly replied.

"Don't be silly," Eduard persisted. "People like Dad should be held up as examples."

"I really don't—"

"I'll contact the college tomorrow," he interrupted decisively.

And the following day, Eduard spoke to whichever body it is that oversees these matters, suggesting that he fund a scholarship, established in his father's name, to support needy dental students of Hungarian origin.

Eduard didn't hear anything back about his proposal for quite some weeks, and when he did eventually receive a reply, it was not at all the one he was expecting. Far from praising the idea, the reply made no mention of the proposed scholarship at all but simply demanded that Eduard appear before the dental board to answer a charge of grave professional misconduct.

Eduard was understandably shocked by the letter and went back over every case history for the previous year or so to see if he could find anything that had caused the problem. Unable to unearth anything untoward, Eduard went to his meeting with the board, completely unclear as to the basis of the charge that he faced.

"You are in gross breach of the professional guidelines of the college," said the senior board member coldly to open proceedings.

"But how?" Eduard asked, bewildered.

"By being in partnership with an unregistered practitioner," came the reply, and for a moment, Eduard was struck dumb.

"But that's ridiculous," he said when he could speak again. "I've only ever worked with my father."

"Exactly," replied the chairman of the board. "We had no idea that you'd been in practice with him until we received your letter recommending that we commemorate his services. When college staff investigated your request, they found that he was never registered as a dentist in this country."

"But that's ridiculous," Eduard exclaimed. "He was in practice for almost forty years. There must be some mistake. Of course he was registered."

"I assure you," the chairman repeated icily, "he was not."

"I had no idea," Eduard said quietly after a shocked silence.

"Ignorance is no defense," the chairman said. "This is a serious matter, and the members of the board have already deliberated on it. Our decision is that you be reprimanded and put on probation for a period of twelve months, during which time you will be counseled on the selection of appropriate business partners."

"What!" exclaimed Eduard, and was about to defend himself, but the gavel had come down with a crack and the hearing was over.

"I did try to warn you," Lujza told her son when he returned home, fuming about what had happened.

"You mean you knew Dad wasn't registered?" Eduard asked.

"Everybody knew," she said. "When we came to Australia, your father's qualifications weren't recognized here. We were totally surprised. It just never crossed our minds that they wouldn't be. When his diplomas were rejected, your father provided the board with evidence of all the work he had done in Budapest and Vienna, thinking they would change their minds, but it made no difference. He even presented his folders full of testimonials, but I don't think they even looked at them.

"They said he would have to go back to university and take all the examinations again. He did enroll, but we had you and your brother to feed, and we just couldn't make ends meet. So he threw in his studies and set up a practice anyway. There has never been the slightest problem. Until now," she added.

"What do you mean 'everybody knew'?" Eduard asked breathlessly.

"From the sign painted across the bottom of the front window of the practice."

"What sign?" Eduard replied.

"The one in Hungarian saying 'I am neither registered nor insured so please do not sue me,'" his mother replied. "Everyone who ever came to see him knew that, and not once in forty years was there ever so much as a single complaint. Everyone judged your father by his abilities rather than by any certificates that might or might not be hanging on the wall.

"Your dad and I thought it would make you more Australian if we didn't teach you and your brother Hungarian. Come to think of it, maybe you were the only one who didn't know."

"But—" Eduard started to say.

"Of course," Lujza continued with a smile, "your father put everything in my name anyway, just in case."

▪ ▪ ▪

Only a week or two ago, I happened to be driving past Tamas's old farm, and I pulled over by the front gate for a few moments to reflect on all the wonderful times I'd had there. Eduard runs the place now, and Lujza has moved back to the house in town. I still keep in occasional touch with her, but it's mostly on a Christmas card basis these days.

I stood there in the sunshine for a few moments, thinking of how it all finished up. After the hearing, Eduard's indemnity company lodged an appeal, and eventually common sense prevailed. Eduard's reprimand was wiped from the records, but even to this day, the college hasn't been able to embrace his generous idea of a scholarship.

There were some bunches of daffodils for sale in a bucket by the letter box. In memory of a lovely man, I put the required amount in the tin provided and took some home with me to liven up the kitchen.

RECIPES FOR DISASTER

Risotto Piselli Mais

1 cup rice
1 cup water
¼ packet frozen peas
¼ packet frozen corn

1. Fry rice.
2. Add water, peas, and corn.
3. Heat for a further 10 minutes.

4

SHANGRI-LA

Just to the north of Rushby, at the end of a gravel driveway and behind a neatly kept garden of native shrubs, stands Shangri-La, the old people's home run by Dymphna. Once a week I visit the place to check that all is well with the residents. The visit is always a pleasure, for Dymphna is unfailingly charming, and I am kept liberally supplied with refreshments during my stay.

I normally like to get there shortly after the residents scheduled lunchtime, so as to get my business finished before the arrangements for afternoon tea get under way. On one occasion, however, I was running later than usual and didn't arrive until the residents were already slowly assembling on their sticks and walking frames, heading for the dining room. For once, I was not in a particular hurry, so I sat and had a cup of tea with Dymphna and decided to let the residents finish their refreshments before I saw anyone.

I looked across at the bent bodies and the sea of gray and shiny heads. How easy it would be, I thought, to see them all simply as they were at that moment rather than as they had once been.

"You know," I said, turning to Dymphna, "it's not long ago that this lot were dancing and running and making love and dreaming dreams."

"Yes, I often think of that," Dymphna replied with that lovely sad smile of hers.

And some of the passions and some of the dreams were known to me, for I had been looking after most of the residents for many years, and more than a few of them had shared their secrets with me.

▪ ▪ ▪

In the corner, hunched over her tea and fruitcake, was Doris, who had been a dancer in her youth and who had then spent the rest of her life as a dog whisperer. On the wall of her room, there hung a large hand-tinted photograph of a line of young girls in stage costume.

"Who are these girls?" I asked when I first saw it.

"That one's me," she said with pride, pointing to a leggy teenager. "Paris, 1926. The Folies Bergère," she added.

"Well, well, well," I said softly and leaned forward for a better view.

"I was there when Josephine danced," she said proudly.

"Josephine who?" I asked.

"You know, the naughty one with the bananas. You must have heard of her," she said. "I wasn't a bit like that, of course." She giggled.

But there must have been some similarities, for occasionally the staff would go into Doris's room to drop off clean clothes or linen, only to accidentally interrupt her in the middle of entertaining one of the gentleman residents in ways that clearly pleased both of them.

▪ ▪ ▪

Sitting across from Doris was Marianne, the other half of the French connection, as we called them. Marianne, with her chiseled features, trim figure, and stylish clothing was unmistakably Gallic. She had fought with the French Resistance in the war and then moved to Algiers. Later, when Algeria slipped out of France's control, she and her husband decided to move to Australia rather than go back to Marseilles.

Unfortunately, on the boat out, Marianne's husband was caught *in flagrante* with another passenger, and there was a terrible on-board scandal. The upshot was that the husband went back to Algiers while she arrived in Rushby on her own. And Marianne had lived there ever since, without ever learning so much as three words of English. But if the prophet won't go to the mountain, then we all know what has to happen, and there can be few small country towns where French is so widely spoken by the shopkeepers.

▪ ▪ ▪

At the table next to Doris and Marianne sat Arthur, one of the few that Churchill had felt was owed so much by so many. He had come to Shangri-La after his wife died.

"Without wantin' to speak ill of the dearly departed," he once confided in me, "she was not an easy woman to live with. Hoh, no! Fifty years we 'ad together. Fifty years of marital blitz. Just to let you know how bad it was, there was even a time when I went a full three months without speaking so much as a word to her," he said.

"Good Lord," I said.

"Three months," he repeated with a wry smile. "I didn't want to interrupt her."

But he had certainly made up for this prolonged silence since she passed away, for he had hardly stopped talking ever since.

"Gordon Bennett," he said one day while reminiscing about his early days, "did I get into trouble when the war broke out. All I ever wanted to do was fly, so I recruited me brother into a scheme, and we built this contraption in the backyard. Load of old rubbish it was. Gawd knows where we got all the bits from, mostly from the tip, I fink. Anyway, we eventually gets this fing together, and although it 'ad wings, it would 'ave been stretching it to call it an aeryplane.

"Well, when we'd finished tying it together, we pushes it to the top of the slope behind the 'ouse. I sit in it, and me brother starts the engine. To our surprise, it fired first time, and off down the slope I goes at a hundred miles an 'our. At the bottom of the slope, there was this road with a fence running along the side of it. I fought I was going to plow right into it, but then a miracle 'appened," he'd continued, "and the bloody fing took off."

Arthur stared into the middle distance and didn't say anything for a while, so I prompted him into further recollection by asking how he got back down.

"Oh, that was the easy part," he said. "I 'it a lamp post and fell on a passing delivery van. Luckily, no one got 'urt."

"So what happened then?" I asked.

"Boy, did I catch it in the neck. I got arrested and chucked in the chokey. I was charged with just about everyfing except bigamy. I was up before the beak the next morning, and he gave me a simple choice. 'Jail or the RAF,' he says, 'it's up to you.' So two weeks later, I was flying Hurricanes."

"Blimey," I exclaimed, "how old were you?"

"Sixteen," he replied.

"Did they let sixteen-year-olds have charge of Hurricanes?" I asked.

"'Course not. I lied about me age," he said with a sly grin. "I told 'em I was nineteen. Me dad went mad when 'e found out about it all, but it was too late by then."

"And did you fight in the Battle of Britain?" I asked.

"Yes, I bloody well did," he said. "And I made it through because of fear."

"Fear," he continued, "is what kept me alive. I spent four years looking over me shoulder and shitting meself. Even now, I'm good at backing cars. In them days, the silly sods who weren't frightened stupid didn't last a week. Soon as new recruits arrived for their posting, us old lags could tell immediately if they was going to make it through or not. These days, of course," he continued, "I'd probably have been counseled by some do-gooder, learned to frow all me fear away, not looked over me shoulder, and got meself blown to bloody bits."

"So did you shoot anyone down?" I asked.

"Are you bloody daft? That's what I was bloody well there for, wasn't it?" he replied. "Eight of the buggers I got. I didn't use to fink about them back then, but funnily enough, I fink about 'em more these days. You know, who they were, where they came from, whether they 'ad families, that sort of fing. Never flew after the war, though," he continued, "I lost the taste for it. Even came out here on a bloody boat. Now you've wasted enough of me time, so bugger off."

▪ ▪ ▪

Sitting at the table next to Dymphna and me was Merv, who was a recent arrival. When Merv started having falls, although it was obvious to everyone else that his days of independent living were coming to an end, he got very agitated if the topic was even hinted at. When Charlie, his best mate, as he always liked to call him, died, however, Merv signed himself in within the week.

Merv and Charlie shared, for many years, the smelliest house in Stoney Creek. I visited the place on a number of occasions, and it always took me quite a while to acclimatize. I would try and leave the door open to let in some fresh air, but Merv would always close it after me. Even in winter, you could cut the air in there with a knife. In summer, it was impossible.

"Would you like me to open a window?" I would say.

"What on earth for?" Merv would reply

▪ ▪ ▪

From time to time, the local rabbit population at Woongarra got out of hand, and it wasn't hard to pick when it was happening. I applied the simple rule that if I looked out of my bedroom window of a morning and could see six or more rabbits on the lawn, then it was time to take a firm grip.

"Where are you, Hardy, when I need you," I would mutter under my breath, for the problem had never occurred when he had been around.

In the absence of Hardy, and when the rabbit count hit six, I would go over to Merv's place and ask him to come up with his ferrets for the afternoon. He was always obliging, and within a day or so, he and Charlie would arrive at Woongarra in their battered old purple pickup loaded to the brim with cages full of small furry animals. Charlie would stay in the cab, and Merv would quietly unravel his nets and then enlist my help in putting his little charges down the burrows.

"Now you've got to be careful handling these little beauties," he would say as he held one up, "coz I've starved 'em since yesterday to make 'em work a bit harder."

But as careful as I was, I don't think there was ever a time that I didn't get bitten.

On one of his ferreting visits, my mother happened to be staying up for the weekend. Usually Merv left as soon as he had finished all the burrows, but this time I couldn't get rid of him. First, he stayed on for a cup of tea, and then he invited himself for dinner.

"Fine-looking woman, that mother of yours," he confided in me later, and with some cosmic insight not obvious to the casual observer, he would magically appear every time my mother came up from town, bringing with him baskets of mushrooms or tomatoes or bok choy for her.

"What's bok choy?" my mother asked him.

"I'm sorry," Merv answered. "You'll have to speak up. I'm deaf in one ear, and I can't hear out of the other one."

Nothing ever came of Merv's infatuation, of course. "I'm sure he's a lovely man," my mother would say, "but he does have a distinct odor. What is it, by the way?"

"Mostly ferrets and issues relating to personal hygiene," I would reply. "And also sharing his life with Charlie," I added, for Merv had never been able to teach Charlie even the basic rudiments of either house training or car training.

There had been a time when Merv had kept an old ewe at the back of his house. "To keep the weeds down," he used to say. Obviously, she had also entertained a woolly visitor for, one vile winter's night, and totally unexpectedly, she presented Merv with a lamb and then promptly died from the effort of it all. Feeling sorry for the poor little thing being out in the cold and the wet, Merv brought the lamb indoors and fed it with milk from an old beer bottle. And indoors, Charlie had stayed ever since. Over time, he grew until he could hardly get out of the door anymore, and he would just lie down in front of the heater and take up the whole of the living room, or so it seemed. And he and Merv became inseparable companions and lived together for many years until Merv started falling and Charlie went to God.

▪ ▪ ▪

"How are you going for time?" Dymphna asked.

"Not too bad actually," I replied.

"Would you like another cuppa?" she asked.

"Well, I don't mind if I do," I said, and she went off to make it.

Over to my left, sitting on her own in the corner, was Audrey. She had moved into the home when she came out of hospital after swallowing all her tablets in one go. She was always perfectly pleasant to the staff but hadn't really made any friends since her arrival. As I waited for Dymphna to come back with the tea, I cast my mind back to when I had first met Audrey many moons before. It was soon after I'd moved up to Woongarra and only shortly after Audrey herself had moved down from the Hunter Valley. In those days, she lived in a filthy, dingy flat behind the fish and chip shop.

I had been asked to do a house call on her on behalf of Felix, who was busy doing something else, and had gone there during my lunch break. I had found Audrey sitting on the edge of her bed looking dejectedly at the floor. Her greasy hair hung down and hid her face from view. She wore a dirty blue dressing gown that was covered in stains and peppered with cigarette burns. A cigarette hung from her yellowed fingers, and she smelled of alcohol.

"I need a shot for my headache," she said quietly to the floor as I came in.

"Audrey, I'm afraid I don't do shots for headaches," I replied as I cleared some clothes off a chair and sat down. "How about you tell me what the problem is and then we'll discuss what's best to do about it."

"I just need a shot," she repeated without looking up. "If you give me a shot today, I promise I'll never ask you again."

"I'm sorry," I said, "but I don't do shots."

"Please," she begged, but I didn't reply, and there was a long silence. "Felix does," she eventually said.

"I know," I said, and then she started crying.

"You just don't care," she said between sobs. "You just don't know what pain I'm in. Or what I've been through," she added after a pause.

"So why don't you tell me?" I said.

Audrey lifted her head and looked at me for the first time. "How long have you got?" she asked sarcastically.

"As long as it takes," I replied.

There was another long pause. Then Audrey lit another cigarette, picked up a photograph in a silver frame from the bedside table, and handed it to me. It was a picture of a handsome middle-aged man with a beard. She looked at me and said, "Do you know who this is?"

I shook my head silently.

"This is Harold, the love of my life. He was a doctor like you. He was a wonderful and kind man, and I miss him dreadfully."

There was further silence, and then Audrey looked at me again and said, "I was eighteen when I got married. My husband, Jack, had inherited his father's farm, and everyone thought I'd done well. Even my parents thought it was a good match. I wasn't head over heels in love with him, but I liked him well enough, and I'd been tickled pink when he'd proposed. I thought that love would come later.

"Whilst we were courting, he was always the perfect gentleman. He was well-spoken and would hold doors open for me. Every girl I knew wanted their man to be just like him.

"The first time he hit me was the very first night of our honeymoon. We were staying in a hotel. I'd gone up to the bedroom after dinner, and he had stayed at the bar to have a drink with another couple that we'd just met. After a while, I phoned the bar to see when he was coming up and then went to the bathroom to get ready for him. As I walked back into the bedroom, he punched me so hard that he knocked me off my feet. 'Don't you ever embarrass me like that again in front of my friends,' he screamed in my face.

"After that, the beatings became pretty regular. They mostly happened on a Saturday when he got home from the pub, of course, but sometimes they would happen even if he hadn't been drinking. He would flare up over the littlest things, like the wrong meal on the wrong night or work clothes not ironed exactly the way he liked them.

"It went on for years. I don't know why I didn't leave. You didn't in those days, though God knows why. One night, he slammed my head into the washbasin, and that was when the headaches started.

"Eventually, I couldn't take it anymore, and one night I made the big mistake of fighting back. That night Jack really went to town on me, and I finished up in the local hospital with two broken ribs and a face I couldn't see out of. The doctor on duty was Harold, and that is how I met him," Audrey said as she lit up again.

I looked at my watch and realized that I had to be somewhere else. "I have to go, Audrey, but I'll come and listen again if you like," I said.

"Yes, I think I would," she replied. "I'm always at home," she said with a weak smile, so the following week I visited Audrey again. I made us some tea and gave her one of the sandwiches I'd brought.

"Harold's practice was about twenty miles away from the farm," she continued, "but because I liked him, I changed to his practice and started driving over to see him whenever I had a headache. He would even come out to the farm if the pain was too bad for me to drive. Over time, we became quite friendly. Little birthday presents, making jokes. That sort of thing. Bit by bit he told me about some of his life too. His wife was English, and he told me that she hated Australia and made his life hell for bringing her out here.

"Some time later, when Jack was away duck shooting, I had a particularly dreadful headache, and I called Harold out to the house. He was looking especially miserable that day too.

"'Is she giving you a hard time?'" I asked him.

"'She's left,' he replied and started to cry. 'She's gone back to England and taken our daughter with her.'

"He then sat down on the edge of the bed weeping, and I put my hand on his to comfort him. I don't remember exactly what happened next," Audrey continued, "but one thing led to another, and I do know that we finished up breaking every rule in the book."

Audrey paused for a while, smiling at her memories. "It was wonderful," she continued. "He was so kind and gentle.

"We often made love after that. We knew it was wrong, of course, but we just couldn't stop ourselves. We would wait until Jack was away, and then Harold would come over. But Jack must have become suspicious because one day he didn't leave. He drove off as usual but then doubled back and parked his pickup behind the shed and waited.

"When Harold's car pulled up, Jack continued waiting for a while. Then he loaded his shotgun, walked over to the house, burst into the bedroom, and fired from the doorway. As the bedroom door flew open, I screamed at the top of my voice. It was the scream that saved Harold's life by startling Jack and putting him off his aim. Instead of Harold, it was the bedside table that exploded into a thousand pieces. Jack then left, and I've never seen him since. There was a note on the kitchen table. 'Get out, whore,' it said, so I did, and I never went back."

"Wow," I said.

"I can still picture that day very clearly," Audrey said as she finished her sandwich.

"I bet you can," I said and made moves to go. "Would you like me to come back again?"

"Yes," she said, "I would."

"Unfortunately," Audrey said as she picked up the story the following week, "even though the main blast missed Harold, quite a few of the pellets hit him in the back. He bled badly and was in a lot of pain. I bound up the worst of it and somehow got him to Tamworth. I phoned the surgery from there and told them that he was sick and wouldn't be coming in for a while. We then caught a flight to Adelaide and stayed with my sister. Harold had surgery to remove all the shots, and we then found a place in McLaren Vale for him to recover for a few weeks.

"After a while, we returned to the Hunter, and Harold started practicing again. He was busy from day one and often said how surprised he was that not once did any of his patients ever ask about his time off. 'Probably just means that they already knew about it all anyway,' he would say.

"A month later, he asked me if I would stay with him permanently, and I think it was the easiest decision of my life. Sixteen years," Audrey said and paused. "Sixteen wonderful years. That's how long we were together. The best years of my life. He was lovely to me. He cared for me and provided for me and never raised his voice once or so much as lifted a finger.

"I was very much in love, and when Will was born, I thought I would burst with happiness. Never once in all those years did I have even the slightest headache. I thought the good times would just never end. They did, of course," Audrey said with a wry smile, "and funnily enough, it all came about by getting some good news.

"One day, a letter arrived from a firm of solicitors in Sydney asking Harold to attend their offices. They wanted him to sort out some paperwork as a great-aunt had left him some money. He traveled to Sydney a few days later and found that someone who he had hardly even known had left him a fortune.

"At first, we were over the moon about it, but the party came to an end almost before it had started. A secretary at the solicitor's office had accidentally also sent a copy of the aunt's will to Harold's wife in London. She immediately phoned Harold and said that she was returning to Australia to 'collect her due rewards.' She also said that if Will and I weren't off the scene by the time she arrived, that she'd report Harold to the medical board and have him struck off.

"Harold said he would never give in to her blackmail, but in the end, it was me who forced his hand. He was a wonderful doctor and loved by all his patients. There was just no way I could let his career end in disgrace, so I simply left. Whilst he was out at work one day, I put a few things together in a case, got into the car with Will, turned my back on sixteen years of happiness, and never saw Harold again. And this is where I've finished up," she said, looking around at the dirty walls and curtains, "and this is where my headaches came back."

There was silence for a while, and I almost offered her a shot.

"And did Harold's wife come back from England?" I eventually asked.

"Oh yes, she came back all right," Audrey said, "and I understand from the grapevine that she gave Harold ten times the hell that she'd given him before."

"And did he ever try to contact you or Will?"

"No," Audrey said simply. "I imagine that anytime he mentioned us, he was threatened with the board again. When the wife eventually died, some years ago now, I thought about contacting Harold, but a lot of water had gone under the bridge, and I never got around to it.

"Harold's dead now," she continued. "I had hoped that Will would get at least a part of the estate, but the daughter put a stop to that. I didn't even go up for the funeral," she added. "I'm sorry you never met him. You would have liked him."

There was a long pause while we both sat in silence. I picked up the photograph from the bedside table and looked at it again. Even behind the whiskers, I could see Harold's gentleness.

"I wonder what you think of it all," she said as she looked across at me. "We weren't heroes, but we weren't villains either. We were just ordinary people looking for love."

"As we all are," I said quietly, and then to lighten things up a bit, I added, "but there is one thing out of the ordinary. Not many girls can say that a fellow took a shottie up the bum for them," and even Audrey laughed a little.

I was sitting there dreaming about Audrey's story when I became aware that someone was tugging at my sleeve. I looked round and realized that Dymphna was trying to get my attention.

"Hallo," she said, "anyone home? I've got quite a long list for you today, so drink up your tea before it goes stone cold and let's get cracking."

"Would you like to stay on for a meal afterwards?" Dymphna asked as we started our round.

"Thanks, but no thanks," I replied with a smile. "I've already got something lined up."

"I heard you were trying your hand at cooking these days," she said with the hint of a smile. "What are you having tonight?"

"Chicken," I replied.

"Well, don't forget to take the feathers off." She laughed.

"Ha, ha. I'll have you know," I said condescendingly and tapped my finger on her desk, "that these days Gordon Ramsay and Jamie Oliver could do worse than pick up a few tips from me."

RECIPES FOR DISASTER

Pollo Funghi

½ cooked chicken
¼ packet pasta
1 tin mushrooms

1. Boil pasta.
2. Drain.
3. Break up chicken.
4. Open mushroom tin.
5. Mix everything up.

5

GAZZA

If I was to get my love life on track, it seemed that I needed to focus on two things: learning how to prepare a decent meal and having something decent to serve it on. With the help of my friends, I felt that I had now got the former pretty much under control, so that just left the matter of the furniture. *Hand-made would be good,* I thought, and it was while considering how best to resolve the issue that I remembered the timber stacked in the back of the shed in the farmyard.

From time to time, and mostly when I cannot squeeze another thing into them, I clear out the farm sheds. I spend an afternoon taking everything out and dividing it between a "this might come in useful someday" pile and a "one day, I will get around to mending this" pile. I have always planned a "this can definitely be thrown out" pile as well, but it has never amounted to much. Then as the day draws to a close, I put it all back again, just more neatly than before, and justify the entire exercise with the thought that I have, at least, refreshed my memory on the resources I can call upon should the need arise.

During one of these rearrangements, I came across a forgotten stack of drying timber that had been milled from a tree limb that had fallen across the driveway some years before.

I got very excited when I found the timber and, right there and then, pulled it all out of the shed. I then carried it, piece by piece, to the workshop with the intention of immediately making the dining table that I had so often promised myself. I dug up the old photos and sketches I'd made of the table in that Melbourne showroom sometime before and got straight down to work. Evening after evening I went home from the surgery and worked on that project until, after only a couple of weeks, I finished up with a table that looked almost nothing like the piece I had so admired in the showroom. Nothing was quite square, nothing was quite vertical, and nothing was quite horizontal. When you leaned on it, it rocked a little, and there were gaps in some of the joints. In all truth, I was bit disappointed with the final result and left it in the workshop.

It was at about this same time that I started visiting Jack, who lived out on the Folger Road in a falling-down weatherboard encircled by several acres of rusting Volkswagens. Jack, who had become far too frail to visit the surgery, had a spectacular list of respiratory problems and, since he failed to see the slightest connection between not being able to breathe and smoking fifty cigarettes a day, proved to be an uphill battle from a medical point of view.

"My father was a heavy smoker," he would say, "and his father before him, and they both lived into their nineties."

Although the house was like an ice block, I enjoyed going there. Jack, who invariably wore his Machu Picchu hat and sat under a pile of blankets, looking for all the world like a Peruvian leprechaun, was entertaining company. I would rummage through the mess in the kitchen to find the necessary items for making tea while Jack would slowly peel off the countless layers necessary for me to examine him. Then, when we had finished the clinical side of things, he would regale me with endless stories of dairy farming while we warmed our hands around our cups.

"Tits," he would say. "If you've got healthy tits, you've got everything."

"Yes," I would reply. "I can well imagine you would have. Unless, of course, you're a bull."

■ ■ ■

Surprisingly, and certainly despite appearances, the old weatherboard never did fall down. In the end, it was spared that indignity by an oil lamp which Jack accidentally knocked down the back of the sofa one evening. Jack had had a couple of trial runs at burning the house down with his cigarettes, using his bed and the lavatory as dress rehearsals, but this time he hit the jackpot.

I didn't attend the fire, but it must have been fierce, for I saw the glow of it even from Woongarra. And it was certainly a hot topic of local gossip for quite some time, especially as to how Jack had managed to emerge, completely unscathed, from the inferno. Apparently, he had cheated the fates by the skin of his teeth and had then, with a fireman's blanket wrapped around his shoulders, calmly walked the short distance up the road to his daughter's place. There, together with Sharon and Gazza, his daughter and son-in-law, he then spent the rest of his days amid far more jumble even than he'd left behind, only this time surrounded by an ocean of disintegrating BMWs.

"So what's happening to the old house?" I asked sometime later while visiting him at Sharon's.

"Nothing," he replied.

"Won't the insurance pay for the repairs?" I asked.

"What insurance?" He snorted and looked at his daughter, who turned red. "The money for the premium that was supposed to have been paid by someone not a million miles from here never made it in. It finished up in the slots instead."

"Didn't think Dad would ever find out." Sharon turned to me, smiling her funny little smile. "Didn't think there'd ever be a claim."

And the untouched remains of the old house are there to this day. They are all overgrown now, of course, and there is quite a large tree where the living room used to be, but the old cars are all still there, and the outline of the building is easy to find if you know where to look for it.

Jack never did give up smoking, but unlike his forebears, it wasn't his ticket into the nineties. I visited him on a regular basis at

Sharon's for quite some time until, one night, God intervened and decided that Jack didn't need any house calls any more.

On one of my visits, I remember being surprised to find Jack looking very sheepish and with a large black circle around his mouth.

"What on earth has happened?" I asked.

"Go on, tell him," Sharon said to her father, "tell him what you did. Because if you won't, then I will." Without waiting for her father to reply, she continued, "Smarty-pants here wondered whether fags tasted better if you were using your oxygen mask at the same time."

"You idiot," I said.

"She had a lot more to say about it than that," Jack replied croakily.

▪ ▪ ▪

Sharon's house could never have been accused of being organized or tidy. So much so, in fact, that I had to be careful that all the medical bits and pieces I took around with me didn't get lost among all the debris. In addition to keeping one eye on my possessions, a further complication of those visits was the need to keep the other eye on Poss and Digger, who invariably fought over who had the right to hang off my neck while I examined their grandfather.

But it was a warm and welcoming home, and the tea was always hot. And each time I sat down and pushed aside a pile of laundry or groceries or crockery to make space to write up my notes, I would find myself sitting on a beautifully made chair and leaning on an equally lovely matching table.

"Wow!" I said admiringly when a sideboard also made its appearance one day. "So where does all this furniture come from?"

"Gaz makes it," Sharon said simply. "If you're interested, I'm sure he'd show you his factory."

I said that I'd like that very much, so when Jack and I finished our business, Gazza led me across the backyard and opened the door into a rickety old barn. The barn looked exciting; it sat at a rakish angle to the ground and simultaneously exuded both age and vitality. Once inside, Gazza, built along the lines of a stick insect with an eating disorder, and sporting a wonderful Italian waiter's permanent three days' growth, that I have never successfully been able to master, seemed in his element.

"Used to be a smithy," he said with a gappy grin. "It's listed," he added proudly.

"It certainly is." I nodded, tilting my head slightly.

Inside the old smithy, the place was a confusion of broken furniture, piles of timber, mountains of wood shavings, and what looked like the results of a hundred years of serious hoarding. But none of that caught the eye, for standing in among it all, glued and clamped in various stages of completion, was furniture to die for.

"This is fantastic," I said as I looked around and then glanced through an open side door where, to my surprise, I saw a neatly kept conservatory of lush green plants with serrated leaves.

"The trick," said Gazza, gesturing at the furniture as he closed the side door, "is not to use power tools."

"The trick," I said, "is not to leave the door open when you have visitors."

"The trick," he continued, ignoring my comment, as he gently stroked the top of a partly formed coffee table, "is to do everything by hand."

"Fabulous," I said as I admired the work. "And what's with all the broken stuff?" I asked.

"People bring it in, and I fix it for 'em," Gaz replied simply. "That's what I do. Just like you fix people, speaking of which I must come and see you." And a week later, to my complete surprise, he did.

Since he hadn't been to the surgery before, I decided that I'd better get some background information from him.

"Right," I said. "Let's get down to business. Do you smoke?"

"Oh, yeah, shitloads." He smiled at me.

"And do you drink?"

"Oh, total shitloads," he replied with another smile.

"And do you choof?"

"Oh, *absolute* shitloads," he said with a laugh.

"Well, that's got the general health questions out of the way," I said. "So let's have a look at you," I added and ran the rule over him from head to toe. Surprisingly, everything checked out fine, and with the help of a few tests, I was able to prove that Gazza had better blood pressure, vision, breathing tests, and cholesterol than I did.

Damn it, I thought as I looked at his results, *even his liver is in better shape than mine.*

▪ ▪ ▪

Visiting Jack one day and sitting in the dining room admiring the furniture for the umpteenth time, a brilliant idea suddenly occurred to me.

"How about if I sent a bit of work your way?" I said to Gazza and then went on to ask him if he would fix my table.

"Not a problem in the world, Doc." He smiled back at me through a haze of cigarette smoke.

When I later shared the idea of getting Gazza to sort out my carpentry misdemeanors, all I got from local friends were startled faces and raised eyebrows.

"Really?" they would say. "Do you know anything about him?" they would ask.

"Yes," I would reply, "he has genius in his hands."

"Yes, but do you know anything about *him*?" they would repeat and then share opinions that ranged from the defamatory to the frankly scurrilous. The general consensus seemed to be that Gazza had made a lifelong passion out of failing to do what he should have been doing and had instead spent all his energy doing what he should not have even been thinking about.

"His work is exquisite," I would say.

"Yes but…" they would reply.

And so, ignoring everyone's advice, I invited Gazza over to my place one evening to look at the job in hand.

He whistled through his teeth. "Where the fuck did you get this from, Doc? Excuse the French," he asked as he rocked the table back and forth.

"I made it," I said quietly.

Gazza whistled through his teeth again. He was clearly about to say something, and then he looked up at me and stopped.

"Piece of piss," he said with a kindly smile after a short pause. "Have to be cash of course," he added, "and I'd need something to get me going."

"Not a problem," I replied. "How much would you want?"

"Three hundred," he said without a hint of hesitation.

I blinked, looked at him for quite some time, sucked in my lip, and then slowly pulled out my wallet.

"I'd rather do the table here than take it home with me," Gazza continued as he tucked the money away. "As long as you don't mind me coming and going, I should have it finished in a couple of weeks," he added. "By the way," he continued, "you don't have any food in the house, do you? I'm starving."

"Well, yes, but..." I said and shortly afterward found myself inviting him inside.

"Thanks for the spaghetti," he later said with a big smile as he got into his car. "And thanks for the cash," he added, patting his pocket, and then heading off.

"Well, at least that's got that project underway," I said to myself as a slowly dispersing cloud of blue smoke retreated down the driveway.

Unfortunately, despite his bright and breezy assurances, it was some time before I saw Gazza again. The day he left Woongarra with his pockets bulging, he drove directly to the Swinging Arms, as the local pub is called, got himself legless and then had an argument with a tree on the way home. Fortunately, although he killed the car, he stepped out of the wreckage without as much as a scratch. He then blew an impressive number on a breathalyzer and spent the next little while in a residential home run by the boys in blue.

I initially thought that Gazza might have been treated a bit harshly by the establishment, especially as I was keen for him to get on with my table. It turned out, however, that there were a number of complicating factors, previously unknown to me, including lack of license, absence of registration, loads of priors, and heaps of unpaid fines that had tipped the balance.

I actually thought of visiting him, but I didn't.

"Oh, what a pity," Sharon said, "Gaz would have liked that."

Then late one Saturday afternoon while I was quickly watering the potted plants before heading down to Melbourne to see Helen, Gazza appeared, completely unannounced.

"Hi," I said, "Good to see you. I didn't know you were… back," I added, nearly having said *out*.

"Yeah." Gazza smiled at me. "Sorry I haven't been around. I've been away on business. Thought I'd come over and do some work on the table."

"Great." I smiled back at him. "I won't be here myself as I'm just going out, but you go right ahead."

"Certainly will," he said. "There is just one small problem, however."

"And what's that?" I replied.

"I ran out of fuel halfway up your driveway."

"Are you even supposed to be driving?" I asked.

"Of course," he answered with a wink.

"Oh, in that case," I answered in mock relief, "That's okay. There's a can of fuel in the shed. Help yourself."

"I'm on gas." He smiled.

"So?" I said.

"I'll need towing to a garage," he explained.

"I'm going out," I said.

"Well, in that case we'd better be quick," he said, but it was almost forty minutes before I managed to finally pull Gazza's car on to the forecourt of the Stoney Creek service station.

"Thanks for getting me out of that mess," he said after he'd filled up. "Now you go off and enjoy yourself. I'm going back to your place to get some work done," he said and waved cheerily as he drove off.

I was also about to leave when the girl from the office came out and informed me that Gazza hadn't paid for his gas.

"Oi! Gazza! You forgot to pay!" I yelled after him, but he just continued serenely on his way.

"I don't think he could have heard you," said the girl with a smile.

Despite Gazza's promise, it was, once more, some time before I saw him again, and then it was at the surgery. He appeared one morning looking furtive and carrying a duffel bag. When I asked him what he was up to, he said that he had no idea what I was talking about and that he had simply come in for some eye drops.

"Your eyes look fine to me," I said, and then a head poked out from the top of the bag.

"What do you think you're doing with that owl in my surgery?" I complained.

"Don't be so fussy," he said. "I told you, I just need some eye drops," and on cue, the owl blinked and showed me a pair of red and messy eyes.

I had met Wol before, for he lived on a cat-scratching post in the corner of Sharon and Gazza's sitting room. I am not exactly sure how he came to be there, but I think he might have been hit by a car, lost a wing, and been rescued by Gazza. On my first few visits there to see Jack, I had thought that Wol was stuffed. Then one day, just as I was gathering up my gear to leave, he had blinked. I had nearly fallen over with surprise and had then run inexcusably late because the children insisted on showing me where they kept his frozen mice and how they thawed them out, one a day, to feed to him.

"I didn't say the drops were for me." Gazza grinned.

"I can't possibly give you a prescription for a bird," I spluttered, but for reasons that I couldn't begin to justify, I went and found Wol a free sample from the fridge.

"Here," I said as I handed it across, "though for all I know, this is highly toxic to owls," I added.

Gazza thanked me, stuffed Wol back into the bag, and was on his way to the door when he turned and asked if I also had an eye bath he could have.

"This is ridiculous," I said and went and got him one of those as well. As I was bidding him farewell for the second time, I remembered the table.

"And what about my table?" I asked.

"I'll be getting on to that first thing tomorrow morning," he said, "and thanks for reminding me, Doc, because I wondered if you could see your way to a further small advance?" and to my complete disbelief, I found myself parting with yet another fifty dollars.

Despite the further advance, there was a noticeable lack of activity in my workshop the next day, and the day after, and for many more days after that as well.

When I finally caught up with Sharon, I found out that, far from being annoyed with Gazza, I should have been feeling sorry for him. It seemed that his failure to appear in my workshop was due to factors completely out of his control. Apparently, his reverse gear had blown up, a tree branch had fallen through his windscreen, and a kangaroo had jumped out in front of him.

"And?" I asked.

"And also the police found out that he was driving again," she admitted, and it emerged that Gazza was now attending yet another residential course.

"Oh, and by the way, I never got around to saying thank you," she added.

"What for?" I replied warily.

"Wol's eyes cleared up real quick," she replied.

"So when will he be out?" I asked.

"Very soon," she said, "and when he does, he's told me that your table will be the very first thing on his list," but it obviously wasn't.

"How's your table going?" people would ask.

"Fine, just fine," I would lie.

"Really!" they would reply. "I heard that Gazza was…"

Then one day, getting heartily fed up with forever falling over the table in the workshop every time I tried to do something in there, I decided to store it away. I was about to move it down to the old shearing shed when I had a different thought. I had set out with a particular purpose in mind and was still keen to achieve my goal. So together with all the spare timber, I loaded the table onto the back of the pickup and drove it over to Gazza's place.

There was no one home apart from the dogs, so I opened up the barn, cleared a space for myself, and then unloaded everything. To the top of the table, I taped an envelope with all the drawings and photographs.

I patted the tabletop, had a last glance around, closed up the barn, said goodbye to the dogs, and got back in the pickup.

"Well, that certainly sorted out my love life," I said with an ironic smile as I let out the clutch and headed for home.

RECIPES FOR DISASTER

Red Spaghet

¼ packet of spaghetti
1 chopped onion
1 can tomato soup

1. Boil spaghetti for ten minutes.
2. Drain.
3. Add onions and soup.
4. Heat.

6

BOTANICAL

"Everything going well for you?" I would regularly be asked by well-wishers in the surgery as they winked at me.

"Fine, just fine, thanks," I would answer cautiously, feeling that my personal space had been more than a little invaded.

"Hope you don't mind us asking"—they would smile—"but everyone's saying how much happier you seem these days."

And I was. I had seen Helen a number of times since the dove dinner, and things were progressing well. We had spent some lovely evenings together. Helen may have suggested that she wasn't quite ready for a new relationship, but I certainly was. One evening, at the end of a meal on a balcony overlooking the river at Southbank, Helen had held my hands in hers and done that electricity thing again. I definitely wanted it to continue, so I was delighted when, a few days later, she phoned and suggested a picnic in the Botanical Gardens.

"I'll bring the food," I said.

"Really?" she asked with a touch of apprehension.

"I assume you like coq au vin," I replied, and she said that she did.

It was a perfect late afternoon on the day of the picnic, and for once, I wasn't too far behind schedule. I managed to get away from the surgery more or less on time and, remembering to pick up the food and drink on the way, had an easy run down to town.

We found a space on the lawn by the lake, put down a rug, and spread ourselves out. I dished up the chicken and poured Helen the wine.

I looked across at her bathed in the light of the sinking sun and, for the hundredth time, wanted to pinch myself to make sure it wasn't all just a dream.

That day, however, she was not her usual chatty self.

"You seem a little quiet," I eventually said. "Anything wrong?"

"Well," Helen replied after a pause. "You've heard me talk about my sister-in-law Ginny. I think I mentioned that I went to school with her. She lives in Paris now, and unfortunately, she's not well."

"Oh, dear," I said. "Nothing serious, I hope?"

"I'm afraid it is," Helen replied sadly. "She's had MS for a long time, and unfortunately, it has recently got much worse."

There was a pause while we sipped our wine and nibbled on some drumsticks. We looked at a group of children playing French cricket below us near the water's edge. After a while, Helen continued, "She phoned me a couple of days ago and asked if I would go over there and help look after the children."

"And what did you say?" I asked quietly, not wanting to hear the answer that I suspected was coming.

"Of course I said 'of course,'" she said. "I've known Ginny almost all my life. Of course I said I'd go. The girls are my godchildren as well as my nieces," she continued quietly.

I sat there speechless for a while. "So how long will you be gone?" I eventually asked, unable to keep the disappointment out of my voice.

"I don't know," she answered, avoiding my gaze. "But as long as it takes."

"What, weeks, months?" I asked.

"Maybe."

"Years?"

"Possibly."

"Oh."

"I am so sorry," she said.

"So am I," I replied, trying hard to keep my voice steady. "Is there anything I could do to change your mind?"

"I'm afraid not," she replied. "I'm so sorry, Paul, but I fly out on Sunday."

I sat in stunned silence, looking unseeingly at the manicured gardens around us. I was devastated, and it took me a while to hide my emotions.

"But what about your brother?" I eventually asked. "Why can't he look after his own children?"

"Well, he hasn't so far," Helen replied, "and it doesn't look as if he's going to do so anytime soon."

With a shaking hand, I refilled our glasses. I gulped down the contents of mine and thought dark thoughts of Helen's brother. It was he who had largely created this situation by running off with one of his nursing staff.

Helen's brother might be good at poking telescopes up people's bums, I thought, *but he doesn't seem to know a lot about much else. Bloody surgeons.*

I was thinking about which bits of him I'd like to poke a telescope into when I became aware that Helen was speaking to me again. She was asking me for a favor.

"There is one small thing which I'd love you to do for me while I'm away," she said as she put her hand on mine, but this time there was no electric charge at all.

"And what is that?" I said dully.

"I wonder," she said, "if, while I'm gone, you'd look after Chanel for me." It took me a little while before I understood who she was referring to. "Oh, you mean Her Royal Poodleness, Princess Chanel?"

"Yes."

"You mean that neurotic, pampered, flop-eared French fluff ball you call a dog?" I said tetchily, just to clarify things.

"Yes," said Helen with a nod and a grin, "that's the one."

It had been some while since I'd planted Hardy under the walnut tree, and I really missed having a dog. I had recently thought about getting another one, but not one like Chanel who looked far more like a fashion accessory than something designed for chasing and biting things.

Not that I had been totally dog-less since Hardy died, however, since for a short while I had shared my life with Lucky. Lucky had initially belonged to Ted, an elderly gentleman who lived across from the bakery. When Ted went into acute heart failure one Saturday morning and needed hospitalization, he refused to get into the ambulance unless Lucky went with him. To everyone's surprise, the ambulance crew agreed; and shortly thereafter, Ted and Lucky set off for town together—Ted on oxygen and Lucky on his lap.

How Ted ever hoped to square the situation with the hospital staff on his admission is anyone's guess, but in the event, he didn't have to worry about it. While Lucky arrived at the hospital in rude health, Ted, having passed away near the ring road intersection, did not.

Apparently, upon arrival at the hospital, there had ensued what I believe is known in political circles as a forthright and robust debate. The ambulance officers argued that it was perfectly reasonable to leave the dog with the corpse while the hospital staff saw it in a different light altogether. I understand that although it was Lucky's personal preference to stay with her master, she was overruled by the head of the emergency department, and after her second ambulance ride for the day, she arrived back in Rushby only a short while after leaving it.

On the way back, the ambulance officers discussed what best to do with her. Quite late in the journey, they struck on the idea that she would be ideal for Shangri-La, the old people's home in Rushby. Accordingly, they sneaked in through the back door and left her in Dymphna's office with an explanatory note attached to her collar.

Unfortunately, Lucky wasn't cut out for this sort of work. She stole food from the residents' trays, frequently demonstrated that Ted had never instilled in her even the most basic elements of house-training, and she drew blood from the ear of the resident cat.

Eventually, Dymphna put her foot down and, to this day, I am amazed at how many people immediately agreed with her in recognizing that Lucky was the perfect new dog for me.

"Suit you to a tee," said the nursing home staff.

"A match made in heaven," said Heather and Meaghan.

"Just what you need," said the CWA.

I put up some resistance for a while but eventually surrendered to the onslaught, and one evening after work, I picked Lucky up from Shangri-La and took her home with me.

"Exactly what Ted would have hoped for." Dymphna smiled as she put the dog's bed in the back of my car. "But there is just one thing," she continued, "and I hope you don't mind my mentioning it, but...could you please be nicer to this dog than you were to your last one?"

Sometime before, I had acquired a completely undeserved local reputation for being mean to dogs, and I spluttered with indignation all the way home only to find that Lucky had translated my railing against the injustices of this world into personal criticism and had peed on the passenger seat.

Over the following weeks, Lucky settled comfortably into life at Woongarra and, eventually, even learned where dogs are meant to answer the calls of nature. She was a friendly, affectionate little dog, and we got on well enough; but I was disappointed to find that she didn't know how to talk.

"You're not just Lucky to have finished up here," I said to her one evening as she lay on her back in front of the fire having her tummy tickled, "you're Bloody Lucky."

Then one day, and totally to my surprise, Lucky gave birth to three pups; and unfortunately, the event was not without its complications.

The first complication was that Lucky chose to carry her offspring as far as she could crawl under the floor of the old part of the house and leave them there. The second was that just three days later, she decided to chase a truck delivering feed to the farm, got her tire-biting timing all wrong, finished tangled up among the back wheels, and had herself renamed Dead Lucky.

It was only later that day, however, that the full extent of the problem Lucky had caused came home to me. I was in the office making a phone call when I realized that I could hear some squeaking. At first, I thought it might be rats under the floor, but then with a flash of insight, I realized to my horror that it was hungry pups. For a fleeting moment, I thought of tiptoeing away and pretending that I hadn't heard anything. I even went off and made a cup of tea, but then I brought the circular saw in from the workshop, cut a hole in the floor where the squeaking was loudest, and pulled out three blind pups. Thankfully, I was able to pass them on to Vicky, who breeds Gordon setters and knows about these things.

▪ ▪ ▪

"Earth to Paul," Helen said, touching my arm and bringing me back to the present. "You will take her, won't you?" she pleaded.

"Be delighted," I said without enthusiasm, and the handover was scheduled for when I took Helen to the airport to catch her flight.

The following Sunday morning, I picked Helen up from her home as planned. We were very early at the airport and sat for ages drinking coffee.

"Paul, you're hurting my hand a bit," she said, and I realized how tightly I had been holding her.

"Sorry," I said sadly, "I just don't want you to go."

At the departure gate, I hugged her for as long as I could, but eventually even I realized that the time had come to let her go. I watched her disappear through the barrier and then remained standing there for quite some time afterward.

"Sod, sodderer, sodderest," I said as I turned and forlornly trudged out of the terminal.

Back in the car park, I found Princess Chanel sprawled upside down across the back seat of the pickup, enjoying a short siesta.

"It's all right for some," I grumbled as I climbed aboard, switched on the ignition, and sadly turned for home.

It was just after leaving the airport that I had to suddenly slam on the brakes and pull over to the side of the road. "It's one thing putting up with you being so happy when I'm feeling so miserable," I turned and yelled at the dog as I got out, "but it is quite another when you start farting. Your mistress might have insisted you fly business class on the way here," I continued, "but that was really, really awful, and you're going to travel steerage from now on."

As I opened the back door and reached in to grab her, the princess retreated into the far corner. In a dreadfully affected voice, she said, "On ne voyage pas dans le derriere,"[1] and tried to nip me.

"Yes, well, real ladies don't let fly in other people's vehicles either," I replied tartly, getting my hand out of the way just in time and, with the help of a pair of gardening gloves I found under the front seat, manhandled a very reluctant royal out of the cab and on to the chain on the tray at the back.

It was a breezy journey home, and for much of the time, Chanel stayed huddled up behind the cab, shivering in the wind. Then, when almost home, I looked in the mirror and, to my surprise, saw her standing with her front feet on the side of the tray, her nose in the air, and her lips and ears flapping in the slipstream.

Back at Woongarra, I stopped to check the mailbox and then headed up to the house. I was about halfway up the driveway when my eye was caught by a mob of my deer stampeding in the paddock to my right. I skidded to a halt to work out what was going on. At first, I couldn't see anything at all, but then I saw Her Highness, who must have slipped her collar when I stopped at the front gate, flying along close behind them.

"Come back here, you little bastard!" I screamed at the top of my voice, but I might just as well have been whistling Dixie.

Then to my horror, in the panic of their escape from the dog, the deer got too close to a fence line and a young one went headlong into a fence post. Even from where I was standing, I could hear the snap of its neck. I raced down to the stricken animal, but there was nothing to be done. Furiously picking up a stick, I turned around to teach Chanel a lesson she would not forget, but she had disappeared like snow in the sun.

---

1. I don't travel economy.

Seething with fury, I drove the rest of the way up to the house only to find Chanel waiting for me at the front door, grinning stupidly from ear to ear with her face covered in chicken feathers.

"Que c'est amusant la campagne, n'est pas?"[2] She chuckled.

▪ ▪ ▪

Many years ago, at the end of my first term in senior school, my housemaster had written on my report card that I had made "an inauspicious start." I had been quite pleased at the time having no idea what *inauspicious* meant and taking it to be a compliment. I realized that at least Princess Chanel and I now had something in common. She too had made a start that showed not the slightest trace of auspiciousness but which she clearly thought had gone brilliantly.

In a white rage, I was in the process of telling her what I really thought when she looked up at me.

"Un moment, s'il vous plait,"[3] she interrupted as if I hadn't spoken, deftly slipped out of my grasp, and before I realized what she was up to, squatted on the doormat and emptied her bowels.

"Ah, ca va mieux,"[4] she looked up and said.

I was about to bodily throw her as far as I could when I was stopped by the thought that she'd probably just wander off and kill something else. For a few moments, I pondered what best to do and then had an idea. I locked her in the boiler room and poured myself a whisky. For a while, the plan worked well, and peace returned to my world once more.

At about two o'clock the next morning, however, Chanel finished biting her way through the boiler room door, escaped, found the chook bin under the sink, and feasted on the leftovers of the coq au vin. She then regurgitated them all over the floor, climbed onto the couch, and kicked back for a bit of shut-eye.

---

2. Isn't the countryside a hoot?
3. Excuse me for a moment, please.
4. Ah, that feels better.

Fretting that, hour by hour, Helen and I were getting about as far apart as you can get on this planet, I slept badly that night and got up around three to make myself a cup of tea. After I cleaned the dog vomit from my foot, I pulled Her Highness off the couch and sat down on it myself. I was thinking how hard done by I was when Chanel looked up at me with that pointy black face of hers.

"Aujourd'hui," she said, "etait un jour inoubliable."[5]

"Ain't that the truth." I sighed with sagging shoulders. "But why, for God's sake," I added, "can't you at least speak in English like a normal dog?" I finished my tea, threatened violence if there were any further misdemeanors, turned out the lights, and was on my way back to bed when the phone rang.

It was Helen to let me know that she was in Dubai and wanting to find out how Chanel was settling in.

There was a long pause while I considered listing the day's events, but then my shoulders dropped. "Fine, just fine," I eventually said.

"Oh, thank goodness for that." Helen sighed with relief. "I just knew the two of you would get along."

5. Today has been totally unforgettable.

RECIPES FOR DISASTER

Coq Au Vin

½ charcoal chicken
1 bottle Sauvignon blanc

1. Call into the chicken shop.
2. Call into the bottle shop.
3. Go straight to the botanical gardens.

7

RUBY

With the arrival of winter, the workload in the practice rose dramatically. Poor Leslie, our practice nurse who looked after all the "walk-ins," was in danger of being swamped by the deluge, and we looked around for someone to give her a hand. We tried a couple of the locals, but they didn't work out. I'm not sure what the problem was. Either they weren't right for us, or we weren't right for them.

"You know just about everyone around," Meaghan said to me at lunch one day. "Surely you can think of someone suitable."

"Not really," I replied and then had a flash of inspiration. "Well, actually, I do know of someone. She's completely inexperienced and needs to stay close to her oxygen cylinder, but apart from that she's perfect," I said. "And I know she'll be qualified because on Thursday night, I'm going to her graduation."

And Thursday night was delightful. I had never been to a graduation in a football stadium before and rather enjoyed it. The various faculties of the university were arranged around the playing surface, like segments of a cake, and the stands were packed with family and well-wishers. Everyone clapped as names were read out, and different sections of the crowd cheered loudly when loved ones went up to receive their degrees. Then, when all the certificates had been presented, a rock band started playing to some strobe lights, and I wended my way down on to the playing field together with Kat, the mother of the new graduate, to see if we could find the lady in question. There was a terrific crush, and it took us forever.

"Hi, Mum. Hi, Paul." Ruby waved across the crowd when she caught sight of us.

"Congratulations, Nurse Ruby," we said when we eventually got within hugging distance.

"So what are you planning to do next?" I asked her over coffee a little later, expecting her to talk about her career.

"Well," she said, "as soon as you guys leave, I'm catching up with some friends and I'm going to get shit-faced."

"But just remember that in the morning you'll be sober," I said in what I thought was a witty misquote, but she just looked at me blankly. "But before you cover your face in excrement," I continued, "I have a job offer for you. Why not come and work at the practice?"

▪ ▪ ▪

Ruby was four when we first met for the first time. She had fallen off her bike and made a horrible mess of her face. She likes to tell everyone that I threatened to break her arms if she didn't keep still while I stitched up her eyebrow. I don't remember that at all, but if it is true, then it obviously worked, for these days she can't even remember which side she landed on.

She started school the following year, and it became immediately obvious to her teachers, as it had long been to the rest of us, that Ruby was a very gifted girl indeed. Be it in math or running or English or painting, she was a star, and the teachers rightly decided that she should be moved into the acceleration stream at the start of the following term.

Unfortunately, that didn't happen, and for the simple reason that Ruby never even made it back to school after the holidays. She fell ill over the Easter break and spent most of the rest of the year in hospital.

Although it had never stopped her from being bright and bubbly, Ruby had been unwell on and off ever since I had known her and was forever attending the surgery with yet another chest infection. Often she would have a course of antibiotics and then, just a short time later, be back again, needing yet more. Although she only ever came to see me when she was ill, I enjoyed seeing her. Even then, she was unfailingly chatty and always had a drawing or something she'd made as a present for me.

After a particularly bad winter, I sent her to the children's hospital down in Melbourne to see if there was any underlying reason for her frequent illnesses. The preliminary results didn't show much at all, but then the laboratory dug a little deeper and found that Ruby did indeed have a very serious problem.

Over the next few years, Ruby bounced in and out of hospital like a yo-yo. In the early days, I used to examine her carefully to see if she really did need another admission, but eventually Ruby herself would tell me when she needed to go, and I would simply pick up the phone and make the arrangements.

"I reckon I'd make a good doctor," she would wheeze cheekily. "And I reckon you would at that," I would reply.

Ruby never minded going to hospital. She got to know all the staff by name, and when I spoke to them on the phone, I realized that they were all just as much in love with her as I was.

"She brightens up the place. She's our little ray of sunshine," they would say.

Ruby also got to know all the other children on her ward. "We are a clan," she once told me.

"Clans usually have a name," I said. "What do you call yourselves?"

"The Clever Fellows," she said, and then, in response to my puzzled look, added, "CF, Cystic fibrosis, get it?" and I said that I did.

But while being in a clan and getting close to people is great in the good times, Ruby found that it doesn't work nearly so well when things go wrong. If she ever looked dejected, and I asked her what the trouble was, she would invariably reply that yet another of her friends had gone to wherever our next port of call after this one happens to be.

"There is one good thing, though," she said with a grin one day. "You know how celebrities like to visit the kids' hospital to get themselves in the papers? Well, these days, with almost everyone else gone, Sunday and I have them pretty much all to ourselves."

Then one day, a tearful Ruby told me that Sunday had gone as well. "I know," I said, "I went to her funeral."

"Yes, she said she knew you. I wish I could have been there," Ruby added sadly after a pause, "but they wouldn't let me out of the hospital. I didn't even get to say goodbye to her."

Sunday was the daughter of a lovely, gentle couple in Stoney Creek who were also patients of mine. By unhappy chance, Sunday, like Ruby, was also a Clever Fellow. She had been desperately ill all the way through autumn, managing to hold on only by the finest of fingernails. The first cold weather of winter had tipped the balance against her, however, and her problems had spiraled beyond control.

It was bitingly cold on the day of the funeral. Since the small bluestone church was packed to overflowing, and I was running behind time as usual, I had to stand with a crowd of other latecomers on the lawn outside, wrapping my coat tightly around myself in a largely ineffectual effort to keep out the knifelike wind.

The service was relayed to those outside by loudspeaker, and when it was over, Sunday's classmates came out of the church and lined both sides of the path to the road.

With the appearance of the small white coffin, I had expected to be overwhelmed by sadness, but it wasn't like that at all. As they sang her favorite songs and danced her favorite dances, the children converted a moment of what could have been overwhelming grief into a carnival of joy and celebration. And above them, an entire pod of fat and shiny dolphins, desperately seeking freedom from the ties that held them to the casket, danced and cavorted in the breeze.

One evening, a few weeks after the funeral, I organized to go around after work and have a drink with Sunday's parents to see how they were traveling. I was surprised by what I found.

"We are well," they both said, "and it's because we choose to celebrate the *having* of her, and not get drowned in the losing of her. Come on out the back and see what we've done."

We refilled our glasses and trooped outside to a garden that had been completely transformed since the last time I had been there. The pathways and lawns had all been changed, and in the middle of the garden, shrubs and trees now ringed a large irregular area of paving.

"It looks great," I said, admiring the obvious industry.

"It may be difficult to see from where you're standing," Ron said, pointing to the paving, "but it's in the shape of a heart."

"And so it is," I said, now that I knew what I was looking at.

"Yes," said Jen, "so that whenever we wish to be near her, we can sit out here. Sometimes, when Ron's flying a leg back from Sydney and he's coming in through the Heddington gap, he can even see it from the air."

Shortly after Sunday was tugged along by her dolphins, Ruby fell desperately ill herself and was brought into the surgery by Kat. It was immediately obvious that she needed more care than I could give her, so I organized yet another admission.

"I'm not frightened, you know," Ruby wheezed as we waited for the ambulance to arrive.

"Well, I am, so shut up and just keep breathing your oxygen," I said.

"There are too many things I still want to do," she continued as if I hadn't spoken as she took off her mask again, "and I'm not going to die until I've done them all."

"Well, that's great," I said, "and a good start would be to put your oxygen back on."

■ ■ ■

A few days after sending Ruby off to hospital, I had to go down to town to see my accountant. Since his offices weren't far from the children's hospital, I decided to pop in and see her on the way. She was sitting up in bed, doing some schoolwork.

"Hi," she said with her unforgettable smile as she packed her books away. "I told you I wasn't going to die."

"Well, I'm glad you got that bit right," I said.

"And who's your visitor?" a passing nurse asked Ruby.

"He's my doctor," she replied.

"Oh, sorry, sir," she turned and said to me. "I didn't realize you were on the staff."

"He's not." Ruby chuckled. "He's my *friend* doctor." Then we chatted about this and that for a while, and some kind lady brought me a cup of tea and a biscuit.

I suddenly looked at my watch, realized I was in danger of being late for my meeting, and got up to go.

"I'm the last Clever Fellow left, you know," Ruby said as I reached the door. "I'm the last of the clan, and I've decided on something."

"And what's that?" I asked.

"That I completely *refuse* to die," she said and then after a pause, added quietly, "*You* don't think I'm going to, do you?"

"Well, I know one thing," I said with a laugh, "you've made a wonderful job of avoiding it so far."

▪ ▪ ▪

Why Ruby kept going, when none of her clan mates were able to, remains a mystery. Even now it is not clear whether her continuing survival is due to good management, a quirk of genetics, or just sheer bravado. She wears St. Christopher around her neck, so maybe it has been he who has assisted her continuing voyage, and even enabled her to sail serenely past her parents' separation and the consequent break up of her family.

And through all this, Ruby continued to industriously fill in every possible gap between medical interruptions with schoolwork. It couldn't have been easy for her, and it's a good job she has a twinklingly bright brain in her head, for altogether she spent less than a total of two years in high school.

Against the odds, year 12 was a relatively healthy time for Ruby; and against even higher odds than I can think of, she managed to complete her studies.

As soon as school was over, Ruby told her mum that she needed a break and would like to go and stay for a few days with Katie, a friend of hers who lives over near Ellerstone. Katie gave a parallel story to her parents about staying with Ruby, and then the two naughty fairies hopped on a plane and flew up to the Gold Coast for schoolies.

I understand that initially everything went well, and at least to start with, the girls thoroughly enjoyed themselves. Indeed, they might well have gotten away with the deception altogether if Ruby hadn't tried to impress a group of boys by smoking a cigarette and stopped breathing as a result. She was rushed to the nearest hospital where, after thankfully being brought back to life, someone phoned her mother.

Ruby's reception back home was frosty, to say the least, but it might well have been much frostier still had it not been for the examination results being released the same day showing that she'd done brilliantly.

▪ ▪ ▪

From time to time in the years before the schoolies cigarette debacle, Ruby and her brother Cameron would come over to Woongarra for the day. I enjoyed having the children there, and it gave Kat a bit of a break. She would drop them off in the morning, they would help me out with farm chores during the day, and I would run them back home in the evening or sometimes earlier if Ruby wasn't well.

I loved those days, though getting Ruby around the farm was always a bit of a business since, rather like Mary and her little lamb, there was always an oxygen bottle following on behind.

For a girl who had seen an awful lot of the insides of hospitals, Ruby was initially surprisingly squeamish about some of the farm jobs I got her to do, although it must be said that harvesting deer velvet is not for the fainthearted. Ruby went all pale and wobbly the first time she saw it done, but in no time at all, she was injecting local anesthetic and sawing away with the best of them.

"Don't think that a little bit of blood bothers me," she would say proudly if she got covered. "I'm just glad that it's not mine for a change."

The only mistake I made in entertaining the children was to show them how to drive the Flying Banana, a sort of converted Subaru that I'd bought for the farm when I first arrived in the district. It had no top or windows, and it also had no sides. It became their favorite toy, and they would charge all over the farm in it as soon as my back was turned. With Ruby's cylinder strapped on the back and Chanel wedged between them, they would fly off at a hundred miles an hour. I was terrified in case they would hurt themselves and I got the blame.

"I used to understand Hardy," Ruby said the first time they took Chanel, "but I can't understand a word your new dog says."

"I know," I replied. "I have the same problem."

One day I was fixing something or other up in the yard when the Flying Banana flew around the corner on two wheels, skidding to a halt when the children realized that I was there.

"I saw that," I said.

"You saw nothing." They both laughed and roared off again, scattering the chickens and spattering me with mud.

It was my job to give them lunch, but they didn't think much of my cooking.

"What's this?" they would ask as they prodded their food suspiciously.

"Potatoes."

"We've never seen potatoes done like this before," they would say.

"Well, you have now," I would reply.

▪ ▪ ▪

I keep a small mob of sheep at the farm to clean up all the awkward bits of grass around the farm buildings that are too difficult to mow.

When it was time to get them all in lamb again, I would organize to borrow a ram from Josie and Franco, a lovely Maltese couple I knew from the surgery and with whom I occasionally had dinner.

It so happened that Ruby and Cameron were with me the day I was due to go over and collect the beast.

"This shouldn't take long," I said.

We hitched the trailer to the pickup and, just ten minutes later, pulled into Josie and Franco's driveway. My visit having been organized some days before, I had imagined that the ram might be ready and waiting for us in a pen. Instead, he was lying on his side in the middle of the back paddock with a bag on his head. His feet were tied together with baling twine, and Franco, together with two of his brothers, was sitting on top of him to keep him still.

"Hi." I waved as I pulled up next to them. I opened up the trailer, and surprisingly easily, Team Malta manhandled the ram into it.

"Well, that didn't take long at all," Ruth was saying as we got back into the pickup.

"Thanks for the loan of the ram," I said to the brothers. We waved goodbye and were just about to head off when Pussy Cat, Josie and Franco's daughter, appeared from around the corner of the house and stepped in front of the vehicle.

"My mother has cleaned her house from top to bottom in honor of your visit," she said with a fixed smile. "She has also spent all morning preparing food for you, and you are not going to disappoint her."

So we all got out of the vehicle again and, shepherded by Pussy Cat, went over to the house, sat in the sun on the back veranda and drank coffee and cordial, and ate mountains of Maltese cake and biscuits. I talked about sheep breeding to the men of the family, Ruby chattered away to Josie, and Cameron just couldn't take his eyes off Pussy Cat.

"Your house looks wonderful," I said to a beaming Josie as she brought out yet more food, and Pussy Cat winked at me in appreciation.

"Excuse me," Ruby turned and said to Franco, "but what you did out there is not how Paul loads sheep. And he never puts sacks over their heads."

"There are two ways of doing everything, darling," Pussy Cat butted in. "There's the proper way, like how Paul does it, and then there's the wog way."

"Valentina!" chorused her parents. "Why do you say such things?" but Pussy Cat's only answer was to light another cigarette.

Much later than I had imagined, and feeling overfull with Maltese refreshment, the children and I eventually set off for home. As we were about to leave, Pussy Cat stuck her head through the pickup window to say goodbye. The sun was directly behind her, and her magnificent mane of hair looked as if it was on fire. She kissed both of the children, but when I asked if I could have one as well, she told me to get lost.

"Why is that lady called Pussy Cat?" Ruby asked on the way back.

I was about to say that I had no idea when Cameron, who hadn't said a word all afternoon, quietly leaned forward and tapped me on the shoulder.

"Excuse me, Paul," he said, "but I know exactly why she's called Pussy Cat."

"And?" Ruby and I said in unison.

"It's because she's so beautiful," he said quietly and blushed to the roots of his hair.

▪ ▪ ▪

Despite going to a city university to study nursing, Ruby remained very much the country girl at heart. She loved spotlighting and fox-hunting, and even occasionally brought her friends up to the farm for a clay pigeon shoot. She never missed the Deni Ute Muster, and she attended every *Bachelor and Spinster*, and *Dateless and Desperate* within a hundred miles.

During this time, and despite having a hectic social life, Ruby remained surprisingly well, and there was only one occasion when she finished up in her old ward again.

"You've got furrows on your brow," I told her when she came out.

"Well, I was the oldest one in there," she said, "and it frightened me."

"Good," I replied, "that goes some way towards making up for all the times that you frightened the daylights out of all of us."

▪ ▪ ▪

Although she was well when she joined the practice staff, Ruby's health remained a finely balanced affair. She coughed the whole time and often needed time off, but nobody cared in the slightest because when she *was* there, the place lit up. She also took all the asthma and emphysema patients under her wing and fussed over them constantly. We called her the Lung Whisperer.

The only real problem in having her on the staff was that Ruby took it upon herself to reorganize the entire practice. All of a sudden, everything had a home and a label, and just as suddenly, no one, apart from Ruby, could find where anything lived.

Then one summer's day, Ruby got herself into the evening news. She had been sunbathing by the side of the local open-air pool, when she happened to notice that a child who had jumped off the diving board had failed to come up again.

The pool was crowded at the time, and among all the noise and splashing, nobody else seemed to have noticed. Realizing that the incident had gone unnoticed, Ruby got up and peered into the water. It was hard to see past all the swimmers, but then a cloud fortuitously covered the sun, and she was able to make out the form of a child lying on the bottom of the pool. Without a second's thought, she dived in, pulled the boy up to the side, pumped the water from his lungs, got him breathing again, returned him to his terrified parents, and then went back to sunbathing.

"Fancy putting yourself at risk like that," I said when I caught up with her later after seeing the story on the evening news. "And after all you've been through. I mean why?"

"Because he would have died," Ruby replied. "Duh."

"Well, there is that, of course," I said, "but *you* could have died too."

"Oh, stop it," she said, "and anyhow, who are you to talk? I heard about you pulling Ben from the creek last year."

"That's different," I protested.

"And you can't even swim," she said.

"I don't even know how you heard about that," I replied. "All I can say is that there are a lot of people round here with big mouths."

"Yes, well, I didn't call for the TV cameras either."

Unfortunately, my concerns proved to be not unfounded. Chlorinated water and Ruby's lungs are not a good mix, and two days after she became a hero, she was also admitted to intensive care; and over the following days, her life hung in the balance once more.

I went down to town on one of those evenings and sat with her at the hospital to give Kat a break. Ruby was sleeping when I arrived. After a while, I got up to go; but as I did so, she put her hand on mine.

"Please stay a little longer," she said as she opened her eyes. "I might not see you again."

"What rubbish," I replied quietly. "You've got to get better. Apart from anything else, none of us can find anything in the practice anymore."

She smiled and squeezed my hand lightly and then drifted off to sleep again. I sat looking at her for a while. She was hardly breathing at all; and then, with a big sigh, I leaned forward, kissed her on the forehead, and left.

When I got home, Chanel looked at me with her head on one side. "Comment ca va?"[6] she asked.

"Ruby's dying," I said quietly and poured myself a whiskey.

"Merde!" she said.

"Merde indeed," I replied bitterly.

▪ ▪ ▪

There still isn't a day that goes by that I don't think of Ruby. The practice goes on, of course, but it is not the same without her. I miss her noise, I miss her energy, I miss her cheekiness, and I miss her love.

---

6. What's up?

But I don't miss her with any feelings of sadness, for the night I left her sleeping at the hospital, a miracle occurred. Her lungs started to clear themselves, and little by little, she began to recover. Within a week, she was sitting up in bed, organizing everybody, and within a month, she was home.

"That was a close call," she said when she eventually came back to work, "and since there might not be a next time, I've decided that there's something I want to do and do right now," she added firmly. "You realize that my decision will mean me leaving the practice," she continued seriously, and I nodded, for I had an inkling of what was coming. "But don't think you're getting rid of me for good," she said, "because I intend to come back."

Then she studied harder than she had ever studied before and, just over a year later, got herself into medical school.

"She's very bossy," said a friend of mine on the teaching staff there.

"I know." I laughed. "I think it's what I love best about her."

"Yes," she replied, "that's what we all think too."

RECIPES FOR DISASTER

Pommes de Terre

4 potatoes
¼ tub sour cream
1 bottle sauce of choice

1. Place potatoes in microwave for 1 minute.
2. Break potatoes open and fill with cream.
3. Serve with sauce.

8

PLAYING THE GAME

It was a perfect summer's day. There was a clear blue sky, just the right temperature, and not a breath of wind. I pulled up in the shade of the old oak tree next to the boundary and walked around to the front of the pavilion. I was the last to arrive and was busy saying hello to everyone when Filippo came over to let me know that I would be batting at number four.

Just a few weeks before there had been a fracas in the public bar of the Swinging Arms, the commonly held name for the Dixon's Bridge Hotel. It had all started when Australia, against seemingly insurmountable odds, had dug themselves out of an extremely deep hole and won a test match against the old enemy in Perth.

Apparently, quite a crowd had gathered at the Arms to watch the last few overs on the big screen, and there had been a lot of cheering when the winning run was scored. For a while, there was much good-humored backslapping and buying of rounds, and it was only later that trouble started. It was at around ten o'clock that Filippo, who had kept his views to himself up until that time, voiced what turned out to be the unpopular opinion that the locals had been lucky to win, and had only gotten over the line with the help of some extremely questionable umpiring decisions. He then added, perhaps injudiciously, that he thought it a shame that the tourists hadn't been successful, as it might have taught those arrogant bastards in the baggy green caps a lesson or two.

"And what would a wog like you know about it?" Bluey had apparently inquired and then split Filippo's eyebrow with a quick right jab, ushering in an interlude in which all present felt free to express their views physically.

In response to a call from the barman, I put to one side the stroganoff I was preparing and headed off to Dixon's Bridge.

"Send whoever it is round to the clinic," I had said.

I met Filippo at the surgery just a short while later and set about repairing the damage to his face. As I was finishing my needlework, and knowing that he had no means of transport, I offered to run him home.

About six months before, Filippo had been stopped by the police on his way home from a poker game. He had blown a reading that surprised even Sergeant Hogan and had consequently parted company with his driver's license. Just a month later, he was charged for the same offense while riding his bicycle and, just two months after that, made the same mistake with his ride-on mower.

"What made you want to stir the boys up?" I asked as we got into my pickup.

"A deep love of the game," he replied and flicked his shoulder-length dreads to emphasize the depth of his feelings.

And, as I drove, I heard how Filippo had fallen in love with cricket in Calabria. As a child, he had chanced across it one day on a satellite channel and had become an instant addict. He added that he had seen the migration of his family to Australia as a godsent opportunity for greater access to the sport he had come to adore.

"It's so Italian," he said.

When I raised my eyebrows, he explained himself. "Men dueling to the death with elegance and style. No mercy, no forgiveness, no emotion, and no second chance. And I would like to teach those morons back there," he continued, "that it's not the winning or losing that matters but how you play the game."

"And just how are you going to show them that?" I asked.

"Right now, I have no idea," he replied as I turned into his street, but a moment later, he spoke again. "Yes, I do," he said, "by getting up a team and beating the shit out of them."

"Getting up a team of who?" I asked as I pulled up in front of his house.

"Expatriates, of course," he turned to me and said. "Are you in?"

"Well, yes, why not," I answered. I was going to add that I hadn't wafted the willow since medical school, but he cut me off with a "good" and wrote my name in a notepad that he produced from his pocket.

"I shall, of course, be captain," he announced and got out of the vehicle.

"Have you actually played the game?" I asked.

"Oh yes, Doc," he replied with another flick of his locks. "'Gentlemen versus Convicts'—that's what we'll call it. I'll put the rest of the team together tomorrow."

"Title a touch provocative?" I suggested.

"Perhaps," he replied with a smile, "but I want to grind their faces in the dirt."

"I thought you said it was all about how you played the game." I laughed.

"Of course," he said seriously, "but it's also about knowing which tribe you belong to."

The following morning, I told Heather I had been the first choice to play for the Gentlemen. I had expected her to be impressed, but I should have saved my breath, for all I got in reply were the sort of ill-informed comments that, on reflection, I might well have expected a Scotswoman to make about cricket.

"It'll be fun," I said defensively.

"Aye, well, that's as may be," she said darkly, "but you just watch yourself."

▪ ▪ ▪

"Filippo has done well," I said to myself as I looked round at my teammates, for I admit that I'd had doubts as to how well his team building would go. Although Australia has become richly multicultural over recent decades, I was under the impression that much of this tidal wave of change had bypassed our little backwater. I was clearly wrong.

There was Filippo, of course, and Stef, his brother. Then standing to one side were Costos, wearing mirror sunglasses and heavy gold chain, and Nigel, immaculate in perfect creams.

On the other side of Filippo stood a new arrival to the district who had recently bought one of the local vineyards. He was a tall lanky man who had looked vaguely familiar when I came across him in the practice session, and I had tried, without success, to remember where we might have met before.

He'd had no such problems, however, and came straight over when he saw me.

"Well, well, well," he'd said. "Fancy meeting you again. You used to terrify the daylights out of me," he continued to my complete puzzlement.

"Made my life a complete misery," he announced to the rest of the practice group. "I was a junior at school when he was a senior. 'Spare the rod and spoil the child,' he used to say."

I indignantly spluttered my innocence, but no one was listening.

"The poor bastard travels thousands of miles to escape brutality and oppression," somebody said, "only to find out what a small world it is," and everyone cackled.

And a small world it had recently proved to be, for not long before the day of the match, a newcomer to the surgery had asked at the end of the consultation if I came from Coventry. I was amazed that she could pick it, for I had thought that all traces of my childhood accent had long since disappeared.

"Well," I replied, "more from a small village nearby."

"Which one?" she leaned forward and asked with interest.

"Tile Hill," I said, and she sat bolt upright.

"Tile Hill!" she exclaimed. "Which street?"

"Nailcote Avenue," I replied.

"Oh my god, what number?"

"Six."

"Well, well, well," she said. "I lived at four."

I looked at her for a long while, and then the penny dropped. "So *you* were the Indian squaw who used to climb onto the roof of the pigsty and throw things over the fence," I said in amazement.

"And you were the cowboy on the tricycle," she replied, wide-eyed. There was another long pause while we looked at one another. "You always said you'd marry me," she said.

"Aren't men bastards," I replied, and we both laughed.

▪ ▪ ▪

The rest of the team were made up of Daffyd, a Welshman with the best sideburns in the known world, Alex from Slovakia, Giovanni from the fruit shop, Li from the Chinese takeout place, and Raj, who had recently opened an Indian restaurant, and who was apparently also going to open the bowling. Raj's restaurant had recently won *Best Business* in the local business awards. He smiled as he shook me by the hand and commiserated with me for coming second.

I smiled back at him thinly for I had, in all truth, been mightily displeased. A lot of effort had been put into upgrading the surgery over the previous twelve months, and we had felt confident of winning. At the very last moment, however, Raj's recently opened restaurant had entered the competition, invited the entire shire council out for a complimentary evening meal, and gone on to scoop the pool.

"I told you we should have invited all the councilors in for free prostate checks," Heather had said at the time.

The Convicts were clustered at the other end of the pavilion veranda. I knew them all, of course, and waved a cheery greeting, but they didn't wave back.

They looked like a battle-hardened crew to me, and it was only when I saw them together that I realized what big boys they all were.

A coin sparkled in the morning sunlight, Filippo chose to bat, and the umpires walked out to the middle. When the field had settled itself, Filippo and Nigel strode out and joined them. They went to their respective ends, took guard, looked around at the fielders, and did a few stretches. Filippo then stubbed out his cigarette, and the game got under way.

Although Nigel was out first ball, Filippo and his brother established a good partnership, and I wasn't called upon to bat for some while. I passed the time peacefully enjoying the sunshine on the deck in front of the pavilion and drinking some of the local produce. Even here, though, it was hard not to keep daydreaming of Helen. She had written that Paris was going just fine and that she missed me, but there was no talk of her coming back. There was a number of wives and girlfriends sitting and chatting together in the shade of the oak tree, and I thought how nice it would have been if Helen had been amongst them.

I was still thinking about Helen when my attention was interrupted by a smattering of applause for Stef, who had just lifted a ball into the deep. The applause was, however, cut short when he was given out caught, despite the ball clearly bouncing a good two meters in front of the fielder.

"What!" we all shouted.

"You're wasting your breath," someone said. "That's *their* umpire. But don't worry," they added, "the other one's ours."

"I guess you're on," I heard a voice say, so I picked up my bat and walked out on to the hallowed turf.

I nodded to Filippo, looked round at the field, adjusted my clothing and pads as I'd seen them do on television, and took guard.

The bowler was Rodney, a man I knew well, for we'd spent a lot of time together sorting out his back troubles. Whatever I'd done must have worked, I thought, or he wouldn't be bowling at me right now. I smiled at him as he started his run.

Rodney, spurred on by his recent success against Stef as well as a loud shout from the field of "Give it to 'im Rod," thundered in. His delivery was a thunderbolt, and I didn't get my bat anywhere near it. Instead, it came off the pitch like a swerving red comet and took me just below the left armpit with an atomic explosion of pain and to an immediate chorus of glee from all around.

Rodney, in his follow-through, finished standing right in front of me. "That's for the dog," he boomed.

About a year or so before, while doing a house call on Rodney, I had been forced to defend myself when his dog had attacked me. Fortunately, I had successfully fended the animal off with my foot, but this had led to my being widely, and totally unfairly, branded as a dog abuser. Before I could get my breath back and yet again protest my innocence, Rodney had turned away and taken his hat from the umpire to signal the end of the over.

At the start of the next over, I was able to have some breathing space at the bowler's end for a ball or two, but then Filippo took a run and I found myself facing Bluey. Bluey is a fair bit quicker, even than Rodney, and I never even saw his first delivery to me. I knew it had arrived, however, for it turned my box inside out, and I spent the next few minutes rolling around in agony on the ground to the delight of a ring of laughing fielders.

"That's for my dad's carrots," Bluey leaned over me and barked at me. At first, I had no idea what he was talking about, but then, even through my pain, I remembered.

Marge, Bluey's mother, had told me that she had smoked heavily all her life.

"What, even as a child?" I had asked.

"Probably," she'd replied.

So by the age of fifty, she had developed most of the known complications of smoking and quite a few that hadn't been recorded before. The one that eventually killed her was emphysema, and she spent the last few years of her life sitting in bed at home on oxygen. Not that this ever stopped her smoking, and in fact Marge often said she thought that the best bit about all the medication she was on was that it allowed her to continue puffing for much longer than would otherwise have been the case.

Marge and Joe lived in a pretty Victorian cottage next to the wood mill where they brought up Bluey and his brothers. As she became increasingly immobile, and as her list of medications became ever more complex, I got into the habit of visiting Marge at home every so often to see how she was getting on.

From the road, the driveway to Marge and Joe's place gradually curves round to the house and ends on the lawn next to the vegetable garden. Whenever I arrived, I would say "good morning" to Sally, the Border collie who lived in the kennel by the garden shed, open the gate in the picket fence, and walk to the back door between rows of profuse and magnificent-looking vegetables.

It was difficult to fit in all my house calls, and I often seemed to be in a rush to get everything done. One winter's day, after a week of heavy rain, running late and in a dreadful hurry yet again, I splashed my way up Marge and Joe's driveway at a higher speed than advisable in hindsight. As I came to the end by the lawn, I applied the brakes, but nothing happened. In the heavy weather, the lawn had transformed itself into a shallow lake, and the pickup aquaplaned across it without any obvious loss of speed. I burst through the picket fence, which exploded with a deafening bang, crossed the vegetable patch, and came to a rest near the back door.

I got out more than a little shaken but decided, nevertheless, to proceed with the purpose of my visit. I listened to Marge's chest, adjusted some of her medications, and then had a cup of tea with her. Not one of the family said anything until we had finished, and I was preparing to leave. I was beginning to wonder if they had even noticed the manner of my arrival until Marge spoke.

"Would you like us to leave the back door open next time?" she wheezed. "Then you can come straight in."

"At least the bloody dog is in one piece," Joe said when he came back from checking her. "She's a bit shaken up, of course, but I think she'll be fine." Then he turned to me. "Would you like to drive on through the house, or do you want to reverse back the way you came?" he asked. "There are, after all, a few vegetables you missed on the way in."

"I'm so sorry," I said with a face like a beetroot, "I'll come back later and fix it all up."

"You can't," said Joe with uncharacteristic sharpness.

"Why not?"

"Those carrots were for the Melbourne Show," he said, "the best I ever grew. I'll be lucky if I ever see the likes of them again."

■ ■ ■

When my genitalia hurt no more than my chest, I tentatively stood up again, realizing that I was in a very different game from the one that I'd imagined I was in.

Filippo came down from the other end to see how I was. "How are you feeling?" he asked.

"My chest is on fire, and if I'm ever able to make love to a woman again, it'll be a bloody miracle," I replied, "but apart from that I'm fine. I just want to kill the bastards."

"Good," he said. "I had hoped you'd eventually get the idea."

"I'll show these bloody Convicts," I added and decided that if I was to go down, then I would go down fighting. "The gloves are off," I muttered, and I determined to fight fire with fire and knock every ball out of the park. As a result, the next delivery took the finest of outside edges to the third man boundary, the one after that took the faintest of inside edges to the fine leg boundary, while the final ball of the over went off the extreme toe of the bat high over square leg for another four, making twelve in all.

"Now you're getting the idea," Filippo congratulated me when we met for a mid-pitch conference.

"We have not yet begun to fight," I replied darkly and stormed back to my crease.

That day I flailed like I have never flailed before. The bat is still in the shed somewhere, the center of the blade is in perfect condition, never having been touched, but the edges are all broken away. Perhaps the planets were in alignment, for on that day only two things seemed possible: either I took yet another ball to the soft and fleshier parts of my person, or I dispatched the cherry with the faintest of nicks to the farthest points of the compass.

Then just as I was really hitting my straps, I was given out leg before wicket to a ball that struck my helmet.

"You've got to be kidding!" I exclaimed to their umpire.

"No, I'm not," he said and then went on to express how distressed his aunt had been that I'd written in a book about how she put her night soil on her rhubarb.

"But she does," I shouted down the pitch.

"That's not the point." He smiled back with his finger held high.

When Filippo was run out shortly afterward, having been felled by a fielder in mid-pitch, our innings fell away badly. Our umpire did his best by not allowing a caught behind and by no-balling everything that hit the stumps, but there was only so much that he could do. When Alex, Li, and Con all went in the same over, proceedings came to a halt and everyone went in for lunch.

As the two sides congregated on the pavilion veranda for refreshments, I wondered if dining together might not have been a good idea. Filippo wanted to have a piece of the fielder who'd flattened him, quite a few of the players from both sides wanted to discuss a whole list of issues with the umpires, and I wished to talk to anyone who'd listen about body line bowling. Nevertheless, we did all sit down together, and lunch passed without incident, albeit in an atmosphere that could easily have been cut with a knife.

After the surprisingly liquid intermission, the Gentlemen took to the field, and Filippo and Raj opened the bowling. They were both amazingly good, and after just a few overs, half of the Convicts were back in the pavilion with just a handful of runs on the board.

"Where on earth did you learn to bowl like that?" I asked Filippo as we crossed between overs.

"State reserve team," he answered with a wink.

"No kidding," I said in awe.

Filippo was about to start a new over and was halfway up his run when their umpire held out his arm and stopped him in mid-stride. When Filippo asked what the problem was, their umpire said that, under the rules of this particular fixture, bowlers could only have a maximum of three overs each and must then be replaced.

For a while, there was an extremely spirited debate between Filippo and their umpire about this, especially as no one could remember this particular rule being applied in the first innings. In the end, however, the man in the white coat always gets the final say.

Recognizing defeat, Filippo turned and threw the ball to me, "Okay, Paul," he said, "you have a go."

I took the ball and was about to deliver the first of the gentle off spinners that I had let loose throughout my college years when I suddenly realized that the batsman at the other end of the wicket was Hogan.

I accelerated into the last few strides of my run, aimed straight at his head, and just for once, the ball went exactly where I intended it to. With a loud crack, it bounced off his helmet and sent him staggering back to his stumps to the great acclaim of my teammates.

"That's for laughing when I got hit in the bollocks," I said as he walked off past me. "And also for the speeding fine."

■ ■ ■

A few months before, I had been urgently called out of a morning surgery to attend to Roger, who had collapsed at the tennis club. It had been the final of the mixed doubles. He and his partner were on the point of winning, and it had been Roger's responsibility to serve for the tournament. Unfortunately, the excitement had proved too much for him. He had thrown the ball in the air, but had never even hit it.

When we got the call for help, Lesley and I grabbed the emergency gear, jumped in my pickup, and rocketed off to the club as fast as possible. We worked hard on Roger for some time, but we were not successful. When Roger eventually departed the scene in the back of an undertaker's van, we bade our farewells to all the other players and then, sedately and somberly, returned to the surgery.

Two weeks later, I received a speeding fine. Indignantly, I phoned the police station to explain the situation, but Sergeant Hogan, who had issued the ticket, wouldn't budge. Feeling very sore about it all, I then took the matter to a magistrate's court, but that did no good either. The magistrate upheld Hogan's decision and then gave me a long lecture on the dangers of reckless driving in built-up areas.

"In which case, Your Honor," I replied bitterly, "should I be called upon to attend when your wife has her heart attack, I shall make sure that I strictly adhere to every speed limit."

There was some cheering from the public gallery at this, and I turned and took a little bow, but the only lasting outcome was the doubling of my fine for contempt of court.

▪ ▪ ▪

Unfortunately, for the Gentlemen, the Convicts staged a comeback after Hogan's departure, and no further wickets fell until the scores were level. Things seemed desperate, and then Daffyd walked over and whispered something in their umpire's ear. Unexpectedly, Filippo and Raj were then allowed to bowl again.

"What on earth did you say to him?" I asked later.

"I just let him know that I am fully aware of where he goes to on a Thursday night and felt quite sure that he didn't want it spread around," Daffyd replied with a smile.

"And it certainly seems that he doesn't." I chuckled.

In just a few balls, Filippo and Raj mopped up the Convicts' tail without further addition to the score, and the match, which looked at one stage as if it might have slipped through the Gentlemen's fingers, ended in a tie.

The teams did shake hands with one another as we left the pitch, but there was a lot of glowering and muttering and a general feeling that a number of issues had been left unresolved.

"Are you going to join the rest of the boys over at the Arms?" Filippo asked as I threw my gear in the pickup.

"Well, I wasn't—" I started to say.

"Oh, come on," Filippo said. "Just for once let your hair down—that is, if you had any. It'll do you good."

So I did.

Over the years, I've had little contact with the Arms as a venue for personal recreation. I have quite often patched up patrons from there on a Saturday night, but I hadn't actually been in the place for a social visit since the Christmas in July dinner several years before when I'd won Chaz and his Harley Davidson for the day in the raffle. We visited every winery in the district. It had been a wonderful day but had taken me ages to get over the headache.

"Don't often see you in here, Doc," Bluey said as he came over and shook me by the hand. "Used to see a lot of the fellow who was here before Felix, though. Gawd, he could tuck 'em away. And then when he'd had a skinful, he'd sleep it off on one of them couches over there."

He laughed. "These days, whenever there's a problem, the doc is called out from the surgery to the pub, but back then, it was the other way around. But it was a bloody nuisance really," he added after a pause.

"And why was that?" I asked.

"He kept pet ravens," Bluey said, "and they used to shit all over the place."

"Well, I can promise that I won't do that," I replied with a laugh.

The evening started off in a friendly enough way, and Raj was voted man of the match. Gradually, however, as the evening wore on, good-natured backslapping once more gave way to pushing and shoving.

Then Filippo took it into his head to stand on the bar. "I think you'll all agree," he yelled, "that it's only right and proper that the man of the match should be a member of the winning team."

There was a chorus of cheers and boos, and then someone pointed out that the fixture had ended with the scores level.

"But everyone here knows," he yelled out again, "that we had the moral victory. Everyone here knows that we showed you buggers how to play the game properly."

It was at this point, perhaps influenced by the amount of amber fluid I had consumed, that I made my first error of judgment of the evening by joining in and calling out, "As you would expect gentlemen to do."

There was total silence for just a second or two, and then someone called out, "Go home, you little pommie bastard!"

"This *is* my home," I called back.

"But you're still a little pommie bastard," somebody else shouted and then had a go at me.

It was probably my years of boxing at medical school that then led me into my second error. Without thinking, I ducked and weaved as he lunged, shouted, "I'm as Aussie as anyone here," and caught him with a really good short one in the ribs.

After that, it was pretty much every man for himself.

On a previous occasion, when I had attended a casualty during a brawl in this self-same venue, Bluey had gone out of his way to look after me and protect me from harm. Then when things had finally settled down, I'd asked him what everyone had been fighting about and had been more than a touch superior when told that it was about nothing at all really.

"I think the boys were just letting off a bit of steam," he said.

Unfortunately, this time Bluey was not on my side and didn't protect me from anything. Instead, it was he who, partway through proceedings, pushed a great hairy paw into my face and closed my eye.

As always, however, things eventually settled down. The pushing and shoving reverted back to good-natured backslapping, the furniture was all put back in its rightful place, a final round was shared by one and all, and then everyone went to their various homes, bidding one another farewell and agreeing that it had been a great game.

Standing in my birthday suit in front of the dressing mirror when I got home, I was a sight that would have impressed even Bruce Willis. I had bruises everywhere, my left eye was closed, and my plums were large and purple.

▪ ▪ ▪

"You idiot," Heather said when she caught sight of my eye the next morning and avoided speaking to me until morning tea.

"And what was all this nonsense about if I might be permitted to ask?" she then asked primly.

"I really have no idea," I said after a moment's reflection.

"But what started it?" she persisted.

"I think someone told someone else that his mother wore army boots," I said.

Then when Heather had finished telling me how funny I thought I was, I continued, "Well, we'd just finished playing the game, of course, and everyone was a bit revved up about which side they were on, but I don't really know that it was about anything in particular. I think the boys were just letting off a bit of—"

And then I suddenly stopped, for I realized that I was repeating something that I'd heard once before.

RECIPES FOR DISASTER

Beef Strog

1 steak
¼ packet bicarbonate of soda
1 packet sliced mushrooms
½ tub sour cream
Leftover rice

1. Slice the steak on an angle.
2. Cover it with bicarbonate of soda and water. Heat.
3. Add mushrooms and cream.
4. Serve with rice.

9

CHANEL

After her poor start, Chanel was not allowed in the house. For the first couple of days, she was chained to a tree, but then Heather and Rob lent me an old kennel.

As with Hardy, her diet consisted of offcuts of the meat I had put in the freezer for myself.

"Ou sont mes pépites de poulet?"[7] she asked in disbelief that first evening.

"On this farm, dogs eat real meat," I replied with a smile.

"Le coupe, puis!"[8] she demanded after a moment's hesitation, staring disapprovingly down at the mutton flap I had given her.

"You cut it up yourself, you lazy thing," I replied. "That's what your teeth are for," and although she initially fiddled around for ages, within a week or so, she was at least eating like a dog.

Whenever I got home from work, she was always far more pleased to see me than I was to see her. One day, however, she wasn't bouncing around as much as usual, and I realized that her feet were all swollen. I got out some old clippers and shaved the fur

7. Where are my chicken nuggets?
8. Cut it up then!

off to see if I could get a better view. It didn't really achieve much, so I then took her to see Steve, the local vet.

The waiting room was fairly full when we arrived, and it was obvious that there would be a long wait. It was in this very waiting room some years before with Hardy, my previous dog, that I had been unfairly branded as someone who didn't take care of his animals. I looked around the room and realized that once again I was under scrutiny.

Keen to dispel any doubts as to my dog-loving credentials, I bent down to pick Chanel up and sit her on my lap. Unfortunately, she wriggled at the last moment, slipped out of my grasp, and landed heavily on the floor, crying out loudly and rolling over as she did so.

"Merde!" she yelped, and every head turned to look at us.

"Talk about history repeating itself," muttered the local butcher to the woman sitting next to him.

"And she looks such a sweet dog too," she whispered back.

"Hey, just hang on a minute!" I should have said, and then gone on to explain to them all that Chanel was an abandoned orphan whose mother had gone overseas, and how I'd taken her into my own home out of the goodness of my heart, and what a poor start she had gotten off to, and how much I was missing her mistress, and how difficult I was finding the adjustment.

I didn't, of course. I simply looked away and pretended to study a poster about worming goats while not hearing the disapproving sniffs.

After what seemed like an age, it eventually became our turn to enter the inner sanctum and end the silent inquisition of the waiting room.

"Grass seeds," Steve said after a brief examination and spent the next twenty minutes or so picking them out of her.

"Her feet are far too soft for running around a farm," he continued. "Surely you can see that."

"But…" I spluttered.

"She's obviously a very sensitive little flower, aren't you, pet," he said as he tickled her chin. "What on earth is a little girlie-whirlie like you doing on a big rough farm anyway?" he continued.

"Enfin," she smooched back at him, "quelqu'un qui comprend."[9]

"I understand you just as well as he does," I interrupted. "So can we please move on?" I added, irritated with the pair of them.

"An odd choice for a farm dog," Steve said, "I'm surprised at you. I thought you had more sense." Then before I could explain the situation even to him, he continued, "You'll have to protect her feet, at least until the pads harden up. And next time, please get her clipped by someone who knows what they're doing."

The foot protectors on offer at Steve's practice were a ridiculous price, but on the way home I had an idea, and for the next two months, Princess Chanel walked around in the leather covers from my old golf woods, a relic from some years before when I'd belonged to a swanky club down on the sand belt.

I had started at the club full of enthusiasm to master the ancient sport. Unfortunately, however, my brain and limbs are not wired up in a way that allows for the successful banging of small balls with rectangles of metal attached to the ends of stainless-steel tubes. Consequently, as a result of regular and expensive tuition over the course of an entire summer, I progressed all the way from a natural, if erratic, swing to not being able to hit the ball at all.

I've always thought it a shame for I have only ever had two golfing ambitions. The first is to get around in under a hundred and fifty, and the second is to finish with the same ball that I started with. They are both quite modest, but I have never achieved either of them.

To my pleasant surprise, the idea worked well. The covers fitted Chanel's feet perfectly and were held in place by elastic straps, made by Susie, that crisscrossed over her back—Chanel's that is, not Susie's. I had imagined that Chanel would rail against the idea, but to my surprise, she took to it like a bird dog to water. I think she saw it as haute couture.

When Chanel's coat had grown a bit, I also got Joanie, who does this sort of thing for a living when she's not serving in the post office, to give her an all-over number four, which pretty much got rid of all the silly bits.

---

9. Finally, someone who understands.

"You're sure you don't want any of the pom-poms left?" she had asked.

"Yes, thank you," I'd replied, "I'm absolutely certain."

"Not even on the head and the tail?"

"Especially not on the head and the tail," I'd answered firmly.

And then, because I am not a natural dog brusher, Chanel just grew dreadlocks.

▪ ▪ ▪

Over the next month or so, my new companion seemed to settle into country life. She even eventually reached the point where I would occasionally allow her off the lead during our evening walk.

"Don't think of even *looking* at those chooks," I would growl at her as we walked through the farmyard, "or anything else for that matter," I would add. For a while, everything went well, but then one evening off the lead and with my mind elsewhere, Chanel disappeared on me. I called out, to no avail, and it was only after fruitlessly looking in all the obvious places that I suddenly caught sight of her way off in a paddock. For reasons that remain unclear to this day, she had obviously decided to remind herself what fun chasing deer had been.

On this occasion, however, she came undone through not having done her homework. The most superficial glance at any reference book on deer would have informed her that as the season progresses, they change from the sort of things that Walt Disney makes mushy films about to something more likely found on the set of *Predator*. This time, when Chanel charged at the deer, instead of running away, they charged back. One of them, a little ahead of the others, got to her first. With a flick of his antlers, he lifted her in the air and assisted her to perform a perfect two and a half back somersault with a double twist in the pike position. The only problem being a landing that would not have impressed any judges and caused her hip to dislocate.

Back in Steve's waiting room, I decided, this time, to get in first with the assembled throng. "I guess I just don't know my own strength," I joked with my fellow animal lovers and pointed at Chanel, who couldn't even stand up. Instead of the ripple of laughs that I'd expected, however, all I got was a roomful of raised eyebrows.

Fortunately, Steve was able to pop the hip back in without much trouble, and I was out of there shortly thereafter.

"Paul," he'd said when he'd finished, "there are serious responsibilities to having a dog," but for an answer, I just gave him a withering look.

The sight of the local doctor driving around with a large black poodle with a heavily plastered leg, wearing yellow and green leather boots marked "1" to "4" upside down on her feet in the back of his pickup, completely failed to go unnoticed by the locals. The adults simply laughed, but the children all wanted to climb up and give her a pat.

"Ah, poor doggie-woggie," they would say as they clustered round and fussed over her. "Is your poor leg sore? Are your poor feet sore? Aren't you being looked after properly?"

"Of course she is," I would interrupt. "Now you can all scram."

By the time her hip and feet had recovered, Chanel knew everyone in the district.

"Oohh, ca va mieux,"[10] she said the day I finally removed the plaster and the boots, and for celebration she went for a swim in the lake followed by a roll in the mud under the willow tree. When she had finished, she came back over to me.

"Et maintenant, je tiens à être appelé Nellie,"[11] she announced.

"And why would you want to be called that?" I asked.

"Parce que c'est ce que tous les enfants m'appelent,"[12] she explained.

"Oh, well, in that case, then of course that's what we must do," I replied a little sarcastically and went inside to make a cup of tea.

Over the following months, with all the exercise around the farm, Nellie lost her podginess and bulked up round her shoulders

10. Oohh, that feels better.
11. From now on, I wish to be called Nellie.
12. Because that's what all the children call me.

and rump. In addition, her feet turned into leather far tougher even than the golf covers. An uncomfortable truce settled between us, and as autumn started to wane and the nights began to close in, I let her inside to sleep in the kitchen.

"Just one bite on a door, forage in the chook bucket, vomit on the floor, or sleep on the couch, and you'll spend the winter outside." I glowered at her.

"Ca ne m'a jamais traverse l'esprit,"[13] she replied with a grin.

To my surprise, Nellie stuck to the rules, and I also kept to my end of the bargain. Not that there weren't setbacks and her inexperience with helping with work around the property certainly resulted in a few hard knocks along the way. She was knocked out cold when a fence pole dropped on her head, she was squashed by a mob of sheep in the pens, and she fell out of the back of the pickup when it hit a bump. And with each incident, she would start to make a fuss, then look at me, button up, and just get on with things.

"She's like that Japanese proverb," someone said when I was telling them the story.

"And what's that?" I asked.

"Fall down seven times, stand up eight."

"The really smart thing, of course," I replied, "would be to not keep falling down in the first place."

I got into the habit of taking Nellie along with me when I had errands to run. Though *running* is not the right word, for her presence slowed me down to a snail's pace. We would be stopped every few steps of the way by well-wishers who, ignoring me completely, simply wanted to pat the dog and tell her how cute she was.

"What a great-looking dog," they would say.

"Handsome is as handsome does," I would answer enigmatically.

"So what's she like at farm work?" I would be asked.

"Hopeless," I would reply.

And then someone said, "But she does have *something* going for her."

---

13. The thought never even crossed my mind.

"And what might that be?" I asked a little suspiciously.

"Well, she obviously has the heart of a lion. I've seen how she hangs on for dear life when you're charging round that farm of yours on your motorbike," they said, and everyone agreed.

■ ■ ■

My house is a fair way off the road so that, at least at nighttime, it is usually a very peaceful place. Someone furiously banging on the front door at two o'clock in the morning is guaranteed to get my attention.

"Sorry to wake you," a man I didn't know said when I blearily opened the front door, "but I was just driving past your place and thought you might like to know that there are bulls all over your nature strip."

"Shit!" I said. I gave my Good Samaritan a quick "thank you" and raced back inside to throw on some clothes.

By the time that I backed the bike out of the shed, Nellie was already aboard and holding on tightly to the handlebars.

■ ■ ■

Some months before, Trevor and Bill, two local farmer friends, had talked me into joining a scheme that involved looking after baby bulls. The venture simply consisted of buying calves and then fattening them up until they were ready to be converted into hamburgers for sale in a chain of stores with a household name. The whole thing was financially risk-free, apparently, and would result in such profits that I would be able to spend the rest of my life sitting under a palm tree on some exotic island, drinking cocktails with little umbrellas in them.

In all fairness, the project started well, and fifty bull calves, all missing their mummies, looked cute indeed in the front paddock. The project only turned sour some months later when they all simultaneously hit puberty and, overnight, or so it seemed, turned into testosterone-poisoned teenagers.

When they weren't digging holes, they were bending gates, and when they weren't bellowing or dueling to death, they were planning their escape. However much I barbed-wired and fortified and electrified, it only ever held them back for a few days at best.

I got heartily sick of being interrupted halfway through an afternoon's surgery only to be told that the bulls had got out again.

Heather and Meaghan would hum the theme tune to *The Great Escape* each time I had to leave early, clearly finding the whole thing quite hysterical.

"Just remind us how much money you're going to make out of all of this?" they would ask as I left.

▪ ▪ ▪

I arrived at the front gate to find a gaping hole in the fence and, exactly as my informant had said, bulls scattered over the nature strip, bunting one another in their excitement.

I carefully skirted around to the far side of the mob and then gently started pushing them back toward the hole that they'd made. They were quite reluctant at first, but then they eventually worked out what I wanted them to do. One by one, they turned their heads for home and, to my great relief, slipped Indian file through the gap they had made earlier, as if they had been practicing all week. As I sat astride the bike, watching the procession with relief, Nellie jumped down and went and lay by the edge of the road.

At the moment of triumph, however, with the very last bull about to go back through the hole, a semitrailer, heading north from Stoney Creek, suddenly appeared round the bend. The driver caught sight of me and decided to give me an early morning greeting. As the blast of his air horn rent the night sky, the last bull jumped clear into the air, turning 180 degrees in the process. He then headed off at high speed back toward the road and along what was sickeningly clearly an intersecting coordinate with the oncoming truck. Helpless, I looked on in horror and winced in anticipation of the impending impact.

At the very point of no return, however, the bull unexpectedly skidded to a halt. He then did another U-turn and, to my unimaginable relief, scampered back through the hole to join his mates as the semitrailer raced on, unharmed, into the night.

"Thank God for that." I smiled to myself as I mended the fence with trembling fingers. "How easily could that have ended up in tears?" I added to no one in particular and then called out to Nellie to jump back on the bike for a ride home.

She didn't respond, and when I went looking for her, I found her lying on her side in the ditch by the road, unable to move and clearly in a great deal of pain. It was obviously she who had turned the bull but, just as obviously, not before he had made contact.

By four o'clock in the morning, I was sitting in the casualty department at the animal hospital.

"I'm so sorry," said the duty officer as she came out and showed me the X-rays, "but your dog..."

"No, not *my* dog," I interrupted.

"Well, the dog you brought in has a badly fractured pelvis. She must be one tough ball of muscle to still be here at all," she continued as she stroked Nellie's head. "If she had been one of those pampered princesses we so often see, I doubt that she would have survived. But survive she has, and that means you now have to choose between a really cheap option and a really expensive one."

"What the hell," I said after a few seconds' pause of temptation, "let's go expensive. I'm not sure how I could explain things to her owner if I chose the other option anyway," and Nellie was taken away and pinned and plated to within an inch of my credit card limit.

A few hours later, with the first few pink streaks of a new day starting to show themselves, Nellie was back in recovery, and I was sitting by her trolley and wondering how on earth I was going to get through the day ahead, not having had any sleep. I was interrupted in my thoughts by the duty officer who came in with two teas, sat down, and asked how the accident happened.

"Sounds like you should get a medal, Nel," she said when I finished.

"Yes, I guess I do owe her a thank you, at least," I replied a little grudgingly. Then, when Nellie eventually came around, I carried her out to the pickup and took her home.

"I might now be bankrupt," I said to myself on the way back, "but at least this time I'm going home with a live dog," for on my previous trip to the animal hospital with Hardy, that hadn't been the case.

We were about halfway home when Nellie lifted her head a little and looked at me. "J'aime le nom Nel,"[14] she said.

"I thought you were asleep when she said that," I replied.

"Non," she replied, "seulement reposant mes yeux."[15]

"And I thought that at least one of us had got some sleep last night," I added and yawned widely as I drove on under the ever-lightening sky.

---

14. I like the name Nel.
15. No, just resting my eyes.

RECIPES FOR DISASTER

Pasta in Bianco

¼ packet pasta
¼ cup olive oil
¼ packet grated parmesan

1. Cook pasta. Drain.
2. Mix in olive oil.
3. Sprinkle parmesan.

10

MOTHER'S DAY

Felix and I had always taken turns with weekend and bank holiday duties, but when he had to leave the practice, it left only one green bottle standing on the wall.

My mother, who was still adjusting to being on her own, had readily accepted my invitation to come up for the Mother's Day weekend for a bit of company. I was pleased, for I was getting mightily down in the dumps about Helen's continuing absence, and I needed someone to talk to about it.

While I was looking forward to her visit, it seems that not everyone approaches Mother's Day with the same happy anticipation. A few days before the actual day itself, I was consulted by a man of about my own age from Dixon's Bridge who was clearly depressed.

"What's the matter?" I asked him.

"I don't know if you know," he said, "but it's Mother's Day this weekend. I can't stand it. It's a nightmare."

"But why?"

"Because I've got four of them."

In reply to my look of surprise, he explained that he had a birth mother, a foster mother, and a stepmother.

"And they're all still alive, and they all have to be visited," he continued. "And none of them get on."

"That's only three," I said.

"Oh, yes," he added, "I also have a sugar mother."

"Well, at least you don't have an earth or a surrogate one," I added helpfully.

"There is that," he said, brightening up a bit.

On the morning of the day in question, I served my one and only mother breakfast on the patio.

"Branching out, are we?" she asked, lifting her eyebrows as I put a dish in front of her.

"I've recently got myself a few recipes," I agreed with a slightly superior air.

"Yes, but what *is* it?" my mother asked, poking at her food.

"It's breakfast," I said and moved on to safer topics like her health and how her new vicar was settling in.

"Are you on some health program by any chance?" my mother asked as we finished eating.

"Why do you ask?" I replied.

"Because you've lost an awful lot of weight," she observed, "and you hardly ate two mouthfuls."

"Since Helen's been gone," I replied, "sleep and appetite seem to have rather flown out of the window."

"I like your new dog, by the way," she said, changing the subject. "I never thought you'd get one of those. She's very girly."

I was about to express my views on the matter when I was interrupted by the phone. On the other end of the line, a rather breathless Tanya asked if I could come quickly as her husband, Mike, was lying on the kitchen floor and thrashing about. I pecked my mother on the cheek and, as I shot out of the door, told her that I hoped I wouldn't be too long.

"Very funny," she said from years of experience, "I brought a novel with me just in case."

Mike had been on anti-thrashing-about medication for some years. Although he was very reliable about taking it, he had recently started having a few episodes again. As I flew along, I wondered what the problem could be. "He's stopped now and has fallen asleep, thank the Lord," Tanya said as she greeted me at the door. "But I'll need your help to get Scruffy off him."

It being Mother's Day, Mike had decided to serve Tanya breakfast in bed as a bit of a treat. He had gotten as far as putting the eggs and the bacon in the pan, but had then had a convulsion and thrown it all up in the air. Mike had then fallen on to the floor, and Tanya's breakfast had landed on top of him. He was clearly a crack shot for I have never seen anyone more effectively covered in eggs and bacon.

When the fitting stopped, Scruffy, the family's wire-haired terrier, deciding that it was an ill wind that blew nobody any good, had immediately jumped into action. Not wanting to waste a perfectly good feast, he had hopped on to his master's chest and set to with gusto.

This was not the first time I had seen a dog dining on top of someone. A year or so before, Ray's heart ran out of beats at exactly the moment that he was frying sausages for dinner. Like Mike, Ray finished up on the floor, and like the eggs and bacon, the sausages finished up on top of him. It was then that Pat, Ray's ever-faithful companion, and without doubt the hairiest dog I have ever seen, seized the day. When I arrived just a few minutes later in response to a call for help from Ray's wife, Beryl, Pat looked up at me from Ray's chest with what I think was the head end and said, "Waste not, want not," and I couldn't but agree with him.

I am not sure if Scruffy had ever had a traditional breakfast before, but it had clearly taken his fancy. He was enjoying it so much, in fact, that he was clearly prepared to defend his prize at all costs and snarled at us if we even so much as looked at him.

"He's never done anything like this before," Tanya apologized.

"Don't worry," I replied, "I'm pretty fond of eggs and bacon myself."

Although I was anxious to attend to Mike as soon as possible, I simply sat with Tanya and watched Scruffy breaking his fast. I am a keen follower of emergency procedure protocols, and these always start with a reminder that helpers should never place themselves in danger. As far as I was concerned, this very much included small brown-and-white dogs with pointy teeth and attitude.

Eventually, Scruffy had his fill. He stood up, stretched, belched, and then hopped down for a drink of water. As soon as he did, we sprang into action. Fortunately, it turned out that Mike had been unharmed from either the fit or the fall, and when I had finished checking him over, Tanya and I carried him through to the bedroom and put him to bed.

"Would you like a cup of tea before you go?" she asked.

"I really should be going," I said as I put my gear back into my bag. "I've got my mother waiting for me at home," and then I looked up at Tanya's expression and realized that she really did need a few minutes of my time. "But just a quick cuppa would be fine," I added.

"I recently landed a good job as an accountant," Tanya said as she handed me my cup.

"Yes, I'd heard," I replied.

"My new job pays a lot more than Mike's, and since we don't believe in child care, we decided to do a role reversal. I went out to work, and he stayed at home, did the shopping and cooking, and looked after the kids."

"Very sensible," I agreed.

"We thought so too, but not so some of the locals. People started giving Mike a dreadful time. They slung off at him in the supermarket, at school, everywhere. He was called every name under the sun."

"What!" I said, with disbelief. "Just because he was staying at home? Surely not. I mean, what you two do is none of anyone else's business."

"We know that," replied Tanya, "and you know that, but there are some folks round here whose main interest seems to be commenting on how other people live their lives. I think what pushed Mike over the edge and caused today's little episode was this note left in our letter box a few days ago."

She picked it up off the coffee table and showed it to me.

> Don't come around the school anymore, perving on the kids.

"That's awful," I said. "What are you going to do about it?"

"I don't know," Tanya answered.

"Well, I certainly think you should do something," I said, and I understand that the following day, Mike and Tanya went and saw the headmaster.

He, I am pleased to relate, was every bit as distressed and angry as they hoped he would be and wrote a strongly worded article in the weekly newsletter about bullying.

The culprits were never apprehended, of course, but Tanya has recently told me that they've been left in peace ever since.

■ ■ ■

When I got back home, my mother asked me why I had been so long.

"I had to wait for a dog to finish its breakfast," I said, and she just shook her head.

There were a few other calls that morning, but they were all dealt with easily. Around midday, there was a lull in proceedings, so my mother and I went out for a bite of lunch at a local restaurant.

"I'd like to talk to you about Helen," I started to say as the coffee arrived, but my mother had caught sight of someone she knew and interrupted me.

"Sorry, later, dear," she replied. "Over dinner," and went off to talk to her friend.

There were a several calls during the afternoon but nothing very onerous, and by early evening, the slate was clear. My mother made a meal, I poured us each a glass of wine, and we both sat down.

"I just hope that whoever is in charge of the universe recognizes that no more calls are required today," I said as I sipped my wine. "I have been sleeping really badly recently, and even just one uninterrupted night's sleep would be wonderful."

And with that the phone rang.

"So much for whoever's in charge of the universe." I nodded knowingly to my mother as I reached for the phone. "Dr. Carter speaking," I said in as bright a voice as I could manage and found myself speaking to Edna, a tiny little lady who I knew well from the surgery. She asked if I could come around to her house as George had just died. Edna's husband was a really big man to whom I had often given a lecture in the surgery about his health, and although I expressed my sympathies, I wasn't surprised to hear Edna's news.

"Would it be all right if I came around a bit later?" I said, hoping to have my meal first.

"I need you right away," she replied breathlessly, "I'm suffocating," so I gulped my wine, gave my mother another peck on the cheek, and grabbed my bag.

"I'm so sorry," I said.

"You need someone to help with all this work," she replied.

"Gosh, I hadn't thought of that." I smiled at her and headed out of the door.

"We'll eat when you get back," she called after me.

It was surprisingly difficult to pull George off Edna. Eventually I succeeded, however, and then she found a nightie and dressing gown and put them on.

"Well, I know one thing," I said. "You were lucky you could reach the phone."

"No luck about it," she replied. "I've made sure it's close by for the last year or two, just in case."

We turned George over and straightened him up.

"'Happy Mother's Day,'" Edna said sadly. "They were the last words he said to me. Ah well," she added with a wry smile after a pause, "it was always how George said he wanted to go."

▪ ▪ ▪

Back home and clearing away the plates after our meal, I was about to have another go at talking about Helen when my mother gave a little sob and dabbed her eyes.

"I feel so sad," she said, "being on my own," so we talked about her stuff instead.

"There is also something that *I* would like to talk about," I began to say when we had finished, but I got no further because the phone started ringing again. My shoulders slumped at this further interruption. I counted slowly to three and then went and answered the call.

A man whose voice I didn't recognize said, with just the hint of running his words together, "I wonder if you could come and help. Mother's stuck in the bath."

The address he gave me was in Top Camp, a tiny hamlet tucked way up in the ranges. I had never been there before, but I roughly knew where it was and said that I'd be with them as soon as I could.

It had become a cold and damp night. Even as I reached the front gate, I could see patches of mist, and as I headed up into the hills, the fog became progressively thicker. Between the poor visibility, the time of day, and the fact that I'd not been there before, I traveled slowly. I almost lost my way several times, and it was over half an hour before I drove down a very neat driveway and knocked on the front door of the smallest house I had ever seen. It looked like something out of a children's fairy tale.

After a delay just long enough to make me wonder if I was in the right place, a slightly built man, a little older than myself, answered the door with a glass of wine in his hand.

"Oh, thank you so much for coming," he gushed before I could say anything. "My name's Reggy. But come on in out of the foggy, foggy dew. Mother's stuck in the bath. Would you like a drink?"

"Perhaps I'll see your mother first," I replied.

Reggy giggled, sipped from his glass, and unsteadily beckoning me on with his free arm, led me through a house that was crammed with exquisite antiques.

"What beautiful stuff," I said admiringly as I looked around.

"Well, my dear," Reggy said, "I have always obeyed the first rule of collecting."

"And what is that?" I asked innocently.

"Never, just never, get rid of Georgian," he said.

I nodded wisely and decided there and then that if I ever got around to owning a piece of Georgian, I would never make the mistake of getting rid of it. When I entered the bathroom, having had certain expectations as to what I might find there, I was taken completely by surprise. In my mind, the word *mother* conjures up a certain image. What I found was Hugo, a strikingly handsome man of about my own age.

As carefully as I could, I hid my surprise that there were kinds of mothers I hadn't come across before, and with Reggy on one side and myself on the other, we inched Hugo out of the bath. It was not an easy task, and there was much "oohhing" and "aahhing" from the patient along the way. When he was finally clear of the tub, Hugo was clad in a gown and helped to a sofa by the fire in the lounge, where I checked him over.

"I'm glad to say that I don't think you've done anything serious," I said when I finished my examination. "Your back might be painful, but the problem is simply muscular and will settle down in time. Just take a couple of aspirin and get Reggy to rub it for you."

"Thank you." Hugo smiled gratefully at me. "I feel better already," and I made ready to leave.

"It's bitterly cold outside," said Reggy. "Would you like a little something to warm you up before you go?"

I looked out of the window at the cold, murky night. "I think I will at that," I replied.

Reggy opened a bottle of wine and, with exaggerated care, poured us all a drink.

"So how did it happen?" I asked after a sip or two.

"How did what happen?" they replied.

"Getting stuck in the bath," I said.

"Well," Reggy cut in, "Mother's been getting very menopausal recently, and the only thing which ever pleases him is a new horse, so I bought him one a week ago, and he was exercising it this morning when he fell off. He falls off horses regularly, my darling," he continued, "because, you see, he is simply getting too fucking old to ride them. But do you think he can see this? Of course, he fucking can't. So, in his own stupid, obstinate way, he is not only hell-bent upon hurting himself but also on spoiling my life as well. So there," he added and then drained his glass and poured us all another round.

"Excuse me for speaking for myself," Hugo said, as the drinks were being handed out, "but Reggy has absolutely no fucking idea what he is talking about. This new mare is a little spirited, I will admit, but I came off because she moved sideways whilst galloping—I repeat, *sideways*, Reggy, when the bird gun went off in the vineyard. Have you got that Reggy?" he asked. "When the gun went off, the fucking horse went *sideways*. And in answer to the good doctor's question, I got stuck in the bath because my back went into spasm and was very fucking painful, Reggy, okay, very fucking painful. As you know, Reggy, I have an extremely high pain threshold and hardly ever complain. Nevertheless, you will all be delighted to know that my discomfort is now starting to settle a little."

"What rot, Mother dear," interjected Reggy, "your pain threshold is nonexistent. You don't have one, and there wouldn't be a day when you don't fall off something and complain like a banshee for hours afterwards," he said.

"Boys! Boys!" I said and held up my hands. There was a brief lull in the conversation while we refilled our glasses, and then I changed the subject by asking how long they'd been together.

"Oh god," said Hugo, "since T. rex roamed the world."

"He was rippling with muscles when I met him," Reggy said. "It was at a swimming carnival in Auckland, and I happened to be in the stands. He got out of the water after winning the hundred meters, and it was love at first sight. There was a lot of harrumphing about our relationship, of course, and Hugo was even threatened with being sent back to England."

"Then what happened?" I asked.

"We eloped to Australia where no one cares who you are or what you do, and we set up 'Masai' and make the most delicious children's clothes for anyone who wants to buy them."

"Do you have any here?" I asked with interest, and just a few moments later, Reggy put a pile of tiny dresses on my lap. Even to my completely untrained eye, they looked exquisite.

"Who designs these for you?" I asked as I looked through them.

"What do you mean *who* designs these for us?" Hugo replied indignantly. "Reggy, of course."

"For a while, we did well," Reggy said. "Very well, I mean *very* well. Apartment in Toorak, roller, Tuscan holidays, and Mother Theresa here doing lots of entertaining. But then things started to come in from overseas, and bit by bit, it all slipped away until now, my darling, all we have left is one another and this quaint little doll's house perched on the hill."

"But we won't have even that," Reggy continued after a pause, "if this silly bitch won't stop putting his money on horses that have no idea how to put one fucking leg in front of another."

"I won last week," Hugo interrupted.

"Yes, dear heart," Reggy replied. "But that's just one candle flicker in an otherwise jet-black starless night."

We then toasted Hugo's win, drained our glasses, and refilled them again. "Of course," continued Reggy, who was becoming increasingly difficult to understand, "although we obviously share a bedroom, since there is only one of them in this house, nothing actually happens there anymore."

I was about to suggest that we were drifting into too much information when Hugo cut in.

"This is ridiculous," he said. "Reggy, you are drunk, and if you are going to start saying nasty things about me, then I'm going to bed," and he got up and left.

"As I was saying," continued Reggy as if Hugo hadn't spoken, "The undergrowth no longer rustles. And it's all because…" but there was no end to the story, for Reggy had sunk back into the corner of the sofa, closed his eyes, and had started softly snoring.

Suddenly remembering that I was still supposed to be on duty, I quietly phoned home and told my mother I was on the way back.

"Are you alright?" she said.

"Yes, why do you ask?" I replied.

"Because you sound as if you've been drinking."

"Don't be ridiculous," I replied and accidentally dropped the phone. "Lovely to meet you both," I said to my unconscious hosts and got up to leave. It became immediately obvious that, sometime during the course of the house call, my nervous system had become disconnected from my muscles, and I had great difficulty getting out of the chair. I eventually succeeded, however, and then slowly navigated my way to the door.

The fog was even thicker on the way down the hill than it had been on the way up, and I drove very slowly, keeping to my side of both of the white lines. I berated myself for the stupidly inappropriate thing I was doing and hoped that I wouldn't bang into anything along the way.

"I must be a slow learner," I muttered, for there had been a similar occasion, some years ago, back in London. Half a lifetime before, I had gotten myself legless at the mess party thrown to celebrate our imminent migration across the world. On my way home, I had been pulled over by the police and asked to give my registration number. I told the officers that at that precise moment, I couldn't exactly bring it to mind, but when pressed a little harder, I suggested that perhaps there was an *S* in it somewhere.

"Thank you, sir," they said. "Very helpful. Now where are you going?" I knew the answer to that one, so I said, "Australia."

Well," said one of officers, "who's a lucky boy? You would have been deported for this, but as you're going there anyway, we'll let you off this time. Oh, and by the way," he added, "you'll like Australia. My sister certainly does."

▪ ▪ ▪

I got home to find that my mother had left a note by the phone telling me that she had gone to bed and that there had been no more calls.

"Thank God for that." I sighed. "I'll catch up with my mother about Helen in the morning," I added to myself and dropped into bed and fell into an exhausted and dreamless sleep, which lasted right through until the phone rang half an hour later.

"Hello," I said sleepily, trying hard to swim to the surface. "I'm having difficulty getting to sleep," someone said.

I paused for a while. "And?" I asked.

"Well, you're the doctor on duty, aren't you?" they continued. "I just thought you might have some suggestions."

"Well, as a matter of fact I do," I replied but when I started to list them, whoever it was put the phone down on me.

I had barely put my head back on the pillow when the phone rang yet again. I thought it was my insomniac back on the line and was ready to really let fly. But it wasn't. It was someone asking if I could come quickly to a woman who had collapsed.

I got up and threw on some clothes and was pleased to find that at least my muscles and nerves were talking to one another again.

When I reached my destination, I was initially concerned that my breath might still smell of alcohol, but I needn't have worried. There was a party in full swing, and when I opened the front door, I realized that I was probably in a much better state than anyone else there.

"Where's the patient?" I shouted about the din.

"No idea what you're talking about," said a girl sitting on the stairs and fluttering her eyelids at me, "but why not come over here and play doctors and nurses with me."

She was certainly very pretty, but I declined the offer and eventually found my way through the house to a group of people having a smoke out on the back patio.

"Where's the patient?" I repeated.

"It's me," an elderly woman got up and said.

"I thought someone had collapsed," I said.

"My family came over for a party," she replied, "and now they're talking about putting me in a home."

"And what's that got to do with me?" I asked.

"Well, obviously my mother can only stay on here if there's proper medical cover," interjected an overweight young man wearing chunky gold jewelry. "She said that you'd come if you were called, so I thought I'd put it to the test."

I'm not sure that I have ever been so angry, and I exploded.

"You mean you…" I screamed into his face and then went on to explain to him exactly what I thought about what he'd done.

Apologizing to his mother for my language, I got my point of view across using words that mostly had only one syllable, comprised little more than four letters each, and related almost entirely to human anatomy.

There was a short pause when I finished, and then the rest of the group started cheering.

"Give it to him, Doc," they said. "That was fucking fantastic."

For an encore, I suggested in graphic detail what he could do with his next phone call then just shook my head and left. I was still muttering to myself about the injustices of the world when I got home.

I was about to get into bed yet again when I had a sudden thought and called up my insomniac.

"Hello," came a sleepy reply after many rings.

"It's Dr. Carter here again. I thought you'd like to know that I'm still concerned about your condition," I said, "and was just wondering how you got on with those suggestions I gave you earlier."

An expletive came down the line, and this time it was me who put the phone down.

Fortunately, that was the end of it. Either there were no more calls that night or I slept through them. I got up at first light and made an early breakfast to make sure that my mother and I had an opportunity for a chat.

"I'm so sorry, dear," my mother said as she gulped down her tea. "I don't have time to talk about anything just now. I've got to fly. There's a meeting of the Guild this morning, and I've just got to get back to town. Look after yourself."

"That's exactly what I was hoping to talk about," I replied as I waved her off down the driveway.

Apart from a splitting headache, which lasted for the entire of the following day and made it difficult to concentrate, I thought I covered up the indiscretions of the previous evening well.

"Are you all right?" the patients all asked me. "You look very pale."

"Yes, I'm fine," I replied. "I just had an interrupted night."

"I think it's a bit more than that," Heather muttered behind my back. "He's gradually working himself up into quite a state with Helen being away," she confided in the waiting room.

"I'll be fine," I reassured everyone.

"He's not sleeping, he's not eating, he's losing weight, and he's forgotten how to laugh," Heather replied.

"For goodness' sake, woman. Stop fussing over me," I said irritably and went into my room and closed the door.

RECIPES FOR DISASTER

Breakfast

3 sausages
1 egg
1 cup rice
2 cups water

1. Boil rice in water.
2. Chop up sausages and fry.
3. Break raw egg over them and mix.
4. Serve all together.

11

ANTHONY

The phone rang as I was putting my evening meal in the microwave. I groaned as I went over to answer it, for I felt as if I had done enough for the day, and I was starving.

It had been a day full of delays. Everyone had spent their allotted time talking about minor matters and then, just as they were leaving my consulting room, had turned at the door and said, "I'm sure it's nothing to worry about, and I can see that you're terribly busy and probably don't have the time to talk about it now, but (a) I can feel a lump in my breast, (b) my wife says that there's a black mole on my back, (c) I've been getting some chest pain recently, or (d) There's some blood in my stools. I was tempted to say that I would deal with these matters on another occasion, but one by one I beckoned people back into my room, bid them take their clothes off again, and fell ever further behind schedule.

"I'm sorry to call you so late," Rosemary said calmly, "but we'd like your help. We think something might have happened to Anthony. Could you come as soon as possible, please?"

"What sort of something?" I asked in the vain hope that it could be put off.

"Please, just meet us at his place as soon as you can," she requested.

"Okay," I said tiredly. I turned off the microwave, jumped in the pickup, and sped up to Rushby, only slowing down on the stretch past the police station. Due to the hour, there was very little traffic, and it was not much later that I pulled up outside Anthony's place.

Anthony was a quiet, tall, gangly young man in his early twenties who was polite enough in a detached sort of way. He seemed very much the loner and didn't get himself involved in any of the local activities. I often saw him walking around the town, for although he occasionally found employment, it never seemed to last for long.

I had seen Anthony in the surgery on a number of occasions over the previous few weeks, but at the end of his consultations, I had often felt unclear as to exactly why he had attended. He would present to me with something simple, such as a sore throat, but I could never find anything wrong with him. I often made sure he had the opportunity to discuss what he had really come in for, but he never opened up to me. Although I had seen him off and on for years, I felt that I hardly really knew him at all.

When I arrived at the house, I found his parents standing by the front door. Unlike their son, I knew both Darryl and Rosemary well. Not only were they both regular attendees at the surgery, but Darryl helped fix up the fences on the farm, and Rosemary was well known for the spiritual support she offered to anyone in need of it. Behind them, although the house was in darkness, I could hear laughter and cheering coming from inside.

"Thanks for coming," Darryl said. "We got a call a while ago telling us that Anthony hadn't turned up for a job interview today. He didn't answer his phone when we called him to see what had happened, so we decided to come over. He didn't answer his door either, and yet his television is on. We thought we'd like you here when we went in."

"Of course," I replied. "Have you got a key?"

Rosemary and Darryl nodded. The three of us entered the house and put on the lights.

Anthony was certainly at home. He was in the sitting room sprawled back on the couch. *The Price Is Right* was blaring from the television, but sadly, Anthony wasn't watching the show.

His head was flung back, and he was staring open-eyed at the ceiling. He neither moved nor acknowledged our arrival, and there was a syringe hanging from his arm. The coffee table, in front of him, was a chaotic mess of medications and injections. There was also a rifle lying across it and a half-empty bottle of bourbon.

I tried to protect Rosemary and Darryl by getting in the way of their view. "I had better check him over," I said and attempted to push them back toward the door.

"Of course," they said, but rather than leave, they joined me by his side. "Are you okay with being here while I do this?" I looked up and asked as I knelt by Anthony.

"Of course," they said. "He is our son."

I did what I had to do, but there was never going to be any doubt about the outcome. Anthony had left this world many hours before. Despite the violence of the scene around him, however, he looked completely at peace.

"I'm afraid he's gone," I said, standing up again.

"That's exactly what we thought we'd find," his dad said calmly as he looked down at his son. "How sad."

"Yes," said his mum equally calmly, "this is exactly what we thought we would find. How very, very sad."

"Even as a little boy, he saw himself as a failure," Darryl said. "Despite everything we ever said, he was just never able to see his own worth."

"Sad indeed," I said after a brief pause. I gestured at the contents of the coffee table. "I think we'd better call the police," I added.

Darryl and Rosemary agreed, and a few minutes later, I was talking to the local headquarters. I was originally told that everyone was already out on a job and that there would be a considerable delay before anyone could attend. Without saying whether it had been used or not, I then mentioned that there was a gun involved and was immediately informed that someone would be with us as soon as possible.

"The police are on their way," I said as I put the phone down. "Do you want to stay or go back to your house?" I asked. "I'm happy to wait here."

"That's okay," they said. "We'll stay here with Anthony too," and they sat down on either side of their dead son and put their arms around him.

From the armchair opposite, I looked at them in silent amazement and admiration.

Rosemary suddenly turned to me.

"I am so sorry," she said. "We've been really thoughtless."

"Have you?" I asked.

"Well," she said, "you've been at work all day and probably haven't had time for a meal. Would you like a bite to eat or a cup of tea?"

"Well, that would be lovely," I heard myself answering, and then Darryl and Rosemary got up and went out to the kitchen.

A few seconds later, Rosemary popped her head round the door again. "White or black?" she asked.

"White, thanks," I said.

Then again, a few seconds later, "Sugar?"

"No, thanks."

I sat on my own with Anthony and hoped that the police wouldn't overreact to my mention of a gun.

▪ ▪ ▪

Some months before, an elderly man who was riddled with cancer had decided to end his pain by means of his own shotgun. When the daughter found her father in the garden shed, she had phoned the police and asked them to come straight away. They asked what the problem was, and without thinking to give them any more details, she simply told them that her father had been shot.

The daughter then also called me, and as it so happened, I arrived ahead of the police. As soon as I got there, I went over to the shed to check things out. After finishing a rather grisly examination, I then went back to the house. I was sitting quietly in the kitchen, just keeping the family company, when there was a knock on the door. Since none of the family was in any state to do anything, I answered the door myself and initially thought that there was no one there. Then I looked down and saw Sergeant Hogan in a flak jacket crouched low on the path.

"What on earth are you doing?" I asked, but his only answer was to grab my jacket and pull me down next to him.

"Keep down," he whispered. "There's been a shooting."

"Yes, I know," I replied. "The poor sod's taken his own life. He's over in the shed if you want to see what's left of him."

"Ah," said Hogan as understanding dawned, and we both stood up. "We thought there was some gunman on the loose. Okay, boys," he shouted out, and about twenty armed police rose up out of the bushes. "Nothing doing," he called out to them, and from the looks on their faces, I could see how disappointed they all were.

▪ ▪ ▪

With that, the tea and refreshments arrived. "We're just going home for a minute to let the dog out," Darryl and Rosemary said, "then we'll be back."

Alone again, I sat in the armchair, eating the sandwich Rosemary had given me, and looking sadly over at Anthony.

"What a waste," I said to no one in particular and wondered what would have been needed for things to have turned out differently. In particular, I wondered if there was anything that I could have done.

My mind went back to an evening surgery, some years before, when a young lad of fifteen, who I had never seen before, had come in to see me as the last patient of the day.

In answer to my request as to how I could help him, he initially said he didn't know. Then in bits and pieces, he gradually told me how he had just been dumped by his girlfriend. I listened to what he was saying with one ear, but as he was speaking, I was also thinking wryly back to my own teenage years, remembering similar experiences. When he finished his story, I gave him exactly the sort of common-sense advice and positive suggestions that anyone would give to any teenager who had just had a love tiff. I also suggested that he see me in a few days' time to let me know how he was getting on and then, tired and keen to go home, had sent him on his way.

I did see him again, but unfortunately, it was only a few hours later. At around one o'clock the following morning, he broke into the hardware store and stole a ladder and some rope. He then propped the ladder against a light pole in the high street and tied the rope to the light fitting. It was at about two o'clock when, together with the police and the CFA, I helped cut the poor boy down after a passing motorist raised the alarm.

In my mind, I have gone over the conversation I had with that lad many times. If there were clues as to what was about to happen, I didn't pick them. Perhaps Anthony was the same.

▪ ▪ ▪

I had been gazing unseeingly at the contents of the coffee table for some time, trying to blank out the noise of the television, when I suddenly recognized some of the items on it, and a penny dropped.

Two weeks before, the surgery had been burgled. It had been an amateur affair, but so far, the crime had not been solved. A rock had been thrown through the lavatory window and a hole made in my surgery door by repeatedly stabbing it with a screwdriver. Having gained access, the intruder had then emptied out my drug cupboard and also taken some syringes and needles.

I had no idea if the burglar had been pleased with their haul, but they certainly had gotten away with nothing of any great value. If, before throwing the rock, they had just taken a few minutes to read the notice on the front window, which said "No narcotics or Cash," they would have known that they were likely to be disappointed with what they would find inside. What the burglar did get away with were just normal, everyday injections, and it was these that I now saw on the coffee table before me.

I was sipping the last of my tea when Rosemary and Darryl returned, and the police arrived.

"This way," Darryl said as he ushered the police into the sitting room. There were three of them, and they all stood like statues as they surveyed the scene. Then Rosemary broke the spell and moved toward the door.

"Anyone for tea?" she asked.

"Thanks, but no thanks," they answered and then set about their business. "By the way, does anyone mind if we turn the TV off?"

Nobody minded, so they did, and the laughter and cheering came to an end. "And just for the record," one of them said to me, "he is dead, isn't he? I mean you have checked him over, haven't you?"

"My god, thanks for reminding me. How on earth could I have forgotten to do that?" I thought of replying as three heads swiveled sharply in my direction, but instead I simply said, "Of course."

I have learned not to joke with police when they are concentrating on their work because, only recently, it got me into serious trouble. Not long before this evening, I had presented a talk at a men's evening at the local community health center about the need to maintain health. There had been a terrific turnout, and I had decided to give everyone a few good laughs. I had even told them the one about using two fingers to do a prostate examination, so that you could have a second opinion, and it had brought the house down.

Everything had gone swimmingly well until we were packing up to leave and someone was found collapsed in one of the toilets. We pulled the fellow out of the cubicle and gave him CPR, but it was never going to be successful, and the poor man left in the back of a funeral van.

I had never seen the man before, and since I told the funeral directors I wouldn't be able to sign a death certificate, the police were called in. Two officers duly arrived, and before going home, I was quizzed as to exactly what had happened.

"Did you notice anything suspicious?" one of them asked.

I should have answered no, of course, for I hadn't, but I was buoyed up by a couple of glasses of wine and the success of the evening. In a silly mood, I answered, "Absolutely nothing, apart, of course, from the large Oriental dagger sticking out of his back," which took me months of statutory declarations and further interviews to get myself out of.

Rosemary touched me on the arm and asked if I was all right.

"Sorry, just daydreaming," I said. "Yes, of course I checked him," I repeated with a sigh.

Then the police got down to their detective work. There were calls back to the station to organize forensic experts, and there was an hour or so of taking statements during which more tea was served.

"Do you reckon it takes bravery or cowardice to do this?" one of the detectives asked as he nodded toward Anthony. "I mean, is this gutsy or the easy way out?"

"I don't see it as either," I said. "I just see it as overwhelmingly sad. And maybe also some sort of a crazy, illogical solution to things," I added as I looked over at Anthony's peaceful expression.

"What do you mean by that?" the detective asked.

"Well," I replied, "he may have turned everyone else's life upside down, but *his* troubles are certainly all behind him now."

"The one thing *I* know for sure," said one of the detectives as he sipped from his mug, "is that I've been to plenty of these, and it never gets any easier."

He turned around to Darryl and Rosemary. "Is this your first one?" he asked before I could stop him.

"Yes, it is," they replied quietly as I winced.

"Looks like he was trying to give himself some Dutch courage before doing the job with the gun, and it all went wrong," another of them said.

"I think you're right," I said, indicating the drugs on the coffee table. "None of that stuff is meant to be given into a vein."

"Well, there you go," they all said.

The six of us stood quietly in a circle for a few moments, nodding our heads in agreement with our own private reflections on the evening's events.

"By the way," the senior detective said, "does anyone know where the lad's parents are?"

"These *are* the parents," I said, indicating Darryl and Rosemary.

"Really?" came the flustered reply. "Well then, I apologize to you both. If I'd known, I wouldn't have asked…It's just that you seem so…"

"That's quite all right," Rosemary said. "We understand completely."

"You do?" said the detective.

"Yes," she replied calmly.

The detective looked across at me, and was about to say something else, but he was interrupted by the arrival of the forensic officers and the van from the coroner's office.

There being nothing more for me to do, I gathered up my things and got ready to leave.

"Are these really the parents?" the detective whispered in my ear.

"Yes, they really are," I said, nodding my head.

"Wow," he said. "Is that strength or is that strength."

"It's strength," I replied.

"By the way," the detective continued, "I hope you don't mind me saying this, but I'm hoping you're planning to go straight home and get some sleep."

"Why do you say that?" I asked.

"You look exhausted, lad," he replied.

"Don't worry about me, I'll be fine," I said. "Well, cheerio then." I waved to everyone, and Rosemary showed me to the door.

"I am so very sorry," I turned at the doorstep and said, and a wave of emotion swept over me.

It was some time before Rosemary spoke. "It wasn't your fault, Paul," she said gently.

"Yes, but perhaps…" I replied.

"Paul," she continued, "it wasn't anyone's fault."

"Where *do* you and Darryl get your strength from?" I asked after a pause.

"From being at peace within ourselves. Anthony was never able to do that. At least our poor son is free of his torment now," she replied.

"But how could you both be so calm in there?" I asked.

"Calmness is only ever a reflection of peace in the soul." She smiled at me and said, "And anyway, would our being agitated bring Anthony back? Are you still on your own, by the way?" she continued as we walked over to my pickup.

"Yes, unfortunately, why do you ask?"

"It's just that you don't look well," she said.

"Oh, I'll be fine," I reassured her, "I've just forgotten how to sleep," I said and climbed into my vehicle.

I drove home in a reflective mood and discovered that reheated chicken nuggets taste like pencil rubbers.

"Sont vous okay?" Nel asked as I threw the food in her bowl. "Parce que vous ne regardez pas okay,"[16] she continued.

"No, really, I'm fine," I replied.

Chanel was quiet for a while, and then she shuffled up a little closer to me. "Voulez-vous une cuddle?"[17] she asked, but I told her thanks but no thanks and, being exhausted, went off to bed.

In bed, however, sleep eluded me yet again. I didn't know if it was the wind or possums on the roof or the pipes in the bathroom, but I couldn't even get my eyes closed.

Then there was a knock on the front door, and I got up to see who it was.

To my very pleasant surprise, it was my brother who I hadn't seen in ages. "Mark!" I exclaimed. "What a lovely surprise. How nice to see you. Come on in and I'll make us some tea. What on earth are you doing here?"

"Oh, I just thought I'd drop by." He smiled at me.

"Well, that's very kind of you," I said. "I have been feeling rather on my own lately."

"Yes, that's what I'd heard." He smiled again. "And speaking of that, how's Helen?"

"She's great," I replied. "She certainly seems happy enough. We write and phone all the time, but it's not the same as seeing her, of course, and I'm getting extremely fed up with it all. And worse than that, Helen has recently told me that Ginny is now worse than before, and it looks as if Helen may have to stay on for even longer than she first thought."

---

16. Are you okay? Because you don't look okay.
17. Would you like a cuddle?

"I'm sorry to hear about that," he said, "so why don't you go over and see her?"

"I couldn't possibly leave the practice at the moment," I answered.

"Well, why don't you organize yourself a passport, at least as a start," he suggested.

"Yes," I agreed. "I could certainly do that."

"Excellent," he said. "Oh, and by the way, I agree with Rosemary," he continued. "You weren't to blame."

"But how would you know about..." I started to reply, but I must have drifted off into some sort of sleep, for the next thing I knew it was morning, and I was all stiff and cold in a kitchen chair and Mark had gone.

■ ■ ■

"Were you up all night again?" Meaghan and Heather asked me when I arrived for the morning surgery.

"Why?" I replied.

"Because you look terrible," they said.

I went to the bathroom and had a look at myself in the mirror to see what they were talking about.

"I might have forgotten to shave this morning," I said when I came back out, "but apart from that, I can't see much wrong."

"You need a break, Paul. The practice will survive, we promise you," they begged.

"You know I can't do that," I said. "There's way too much to do here. The problem with you two is that you've been around ill people too long and wouldn't recognize someone who's fighting fit, even if you tripped over them in broad daylight."

12

RITA

There are many different ways of expressing how much trust you should put in other people. My favorite is the one that divides people into two simple categories: those you would go into battle with and those you would not. I would go into battle with Rita any day of any week.

Rita lives up on the new estate, and even by today's generous standards, she is a big girl. She is loud, she is brash, she gets the f-word into almost every sentence, and she could talk underwater with a mouthful of marbles. She dyes her hair purple and is very, very much alive, making it all the more noteworthy that on a recent visit to the surgery, she asked me for the results of her autopsy.

"Biopsy, perhaps?" I suggested.

"Okay, smart-arse," she replied, "now wipe that fucking stupid grin from off your face and just give me my results."

"I have the report right here," I said, looking down at the papers in front of me and then back again at Rita, "and I'm afraid it shows that you have distemper, strangles, pink eye, and hard pad."

"You think you're just so fucking funny," she replied. "Now stop pissing about and tell me what it really says."

"It says that you will live well into the afternoon," I said.

"That's much better," she replied, "and since I've got a bit of time up my sleeve, *and* I'm your last patient of the morning, if you can prize yourself away from that bloody desk of yours for a few minutes, you can come around the corner and have lunch with me," which, since she is good company, I did. I have seen Rita many times over the years, both in the surgery and around the town, but our friendship only really blossomed when we met at Ayesha's home birth. Things were getting a bit stuck for a while, and it was only when Rita bellowed at the mother-to-be to stop mucking about, and push a bit fucking harder, that Ayesha shot out into the world.

Rita is good fun as a lunch partner. She possesses that fascinating combination of a lightning-quick intellect and, having left school at thirteen and paid precious little attention before then, almost no education whatsoever. Life has therefore gifted her with a razor-sharp mind unrestrained by regimentation, and the language skills of a Viking.

She was always a medical disaster waiting to happen. In the event, she didn't have to wait long and her first heart attack came as she was blowing out the candles at her thirty-eighth birthday party. Since then, she's been back to the hospital so often, she says, that they've now given her a key of her own to the cardiology suite and reckons that the only things left to stent are the stents she already has.

"Stop smoking, lose weight, drink less, do some exercise," I would say in my best headmaster's voice, and of course she never took the slightest notice of any of it. Yet for all that, the closest she came to stepping through the pearly gates was when I sent her for a stress test.

"I swear that bastard Paul was trying to get rid of me," she told one and all. "Now," she said at the end of lunch, "you're looking fucking terrible and could obviously do with a bit of feeding up. So get the fuck out of the clinic as soon as you can tonight and come around to my place for tea."

One of the delights of my job is that I am often invited to join families for their evening meal. There is a Maltese family, more or less on my way home, who are particularly kind in this regard. I very much enjoy having evening meals with them. Maltese meals are exciting. Not only does every family member within a twenty-kilometer radius put in an appearance, but the females of the family also spend the entire day meticulously preparing the house for the event.

"What is everyone arguing about?" I asked Pussy Cat the first time I was invited.

"Nothing." She laughed above the noise. "That's just how we all speak."

I was surprised at first, but the answer should already have been obvious to me. Many years before, I had lived next to a Maltese family in London. One Sunday morning, when Mr. Malta was cleaning his car in his driveway, his other half appeared at the front door and handed him what sounded like five minutes of uninterrupted blistering Maltese abuse. When she went back into the house again, I cautiously popped my head back up over the fence and asked my neighbor what on earth he'd done to warrant such disciplinary action.

He looked puzzled by my question at first, but then his expression turned into a smile. "Oh, no," he said, "she was just telling me that lunch is on the table."

▪ ▪ ▪

I've now had tea at Rita's many times over the years, and as with my Maltese friends, it has never proved to be a disappointing outing. Rita always insists that the whole family dine together, so there are always eleven of us crammed round the tiny kitchen table. Apart from myself, there is always Rita, of course; Dave, her husband, who never gets a word in edgewise; and eight children who range from their early twenties all the way down to Colorado, who was still on the boob and very lucky to be there as she'd been accidentally born into the loo.

"How was I to know?" Rita said defensively. "I haven't had a contraction since Dakota."

Rita's pregnancies always seem to take her unawares. She is not alone, however, and I am amazed that the diagnosis so frequently comes as a surprise to so many.

Over the years, I have seen many women who have presented themselves with nausea, weight gain, tummy swelling, and cycle change and who have professed amazement when informed of their diagnosis.

One woman, in particular, I remember who came to the surgery to get something for her upset tummy. As she lay on the couch, ready for me to do an examination, I looked across at her, saw the fetus moving, and started to chuckle.

"What are you laughing about?" she asked, and I told her that there was absolutely nothing wrong with her that waiting for approximately another month or so wouldn't fix all by itself.

"But pregnancy's just not possible," they would all say.

"And just as clearly it obviously is," I would reply.

And if I am amazed that pregnancy can surprise, then I am doubly amazed, as with Rita, that even labor can arrive unexpectedly.

Fairly recently, an extremely pregnant lady asked to be fitted in as an extra on a hectic Saturday morning. When she came into my room, I asked how I could be of help. She answered that she just wanted some antibiotics for a waterworks infection.

"What makes you think you have a waterworks infection?" I asked.

"Well," she replied, "this morning I became incontinent."

"Incontinent?" I queried.

"Yes," she said. "I was standing in my kitchen when there was a sudden whoosh of water down my legs, and now I've gotten some dreadful cramping pains."

But the most memorable surprise was when a teenager was brought in by her mother, having developed severe tummy pains during school sports.

As soon as I put my hand on the girl's tummy, the diagnosis became obvious. I was more than a little shocked and stood silently by the couch for a moment or two, working out how best to break the news.

The girl's mother, who was clearly annoyed at having been called away from her workplace to bring her daughter to the surgery, decided to take it out on me. "You don't even know what's wrong with her, do you?" she snapped aggressively.

"Well, as a matter of fact I do," I replied quietly and asked the girl if it was okay for me to tell her mother. The girl nodded.

"You're about to be a grandmother," I said

"That," the woman said frostily, "is a joke in very poor taste."

"In which case you just sit there and watch while I call for an ambulance," I replied and picked up the phone.

■ ■ ■

"And if you want to know why there are so many little shits sitting round the table," Rita continued, looking over at Dave, "it's because I always took seriously what he pokes at me in fun."

As soon as I arrived for a meal, Dave and the oldest child would be dispatched to the pizza shop, and when they returned, we would all say grace. "Two, four, six, eight, bog in, don't wait," Rita would chant, and the feast would begin. Then when we had finished, we would chat away the evening, sitting in the eye of a tornado of uncompleted domestic tasks. They were wonderful evenings, and although, from time to time, I would suggest that it was my turn to go out and get the meal, I was never allowed to do so. I was once allowed to cook the meal, however, so I made my pork special, which I thought came off rather well.

■ ■ ■

On Wednesday nights, the household program was different. Dave was given full responsibility for running the evening meal, and Rita took the evening off to go and have a flutter. Although she was fond of the ponies, her midweek passion was bingo. I understood that while she usually walked away penniless at the end of the evening, she had recently come home with the jackpot in her pocket and a smile on her face.

"That was a nice win," Rita told me a friend had said to her as she was leaving.

"It certainly was," Rita had replied.

"So could you see your way to lending me some money then?" the friend had asked. "We're a bit behind with the mortgage."

"I told the cheeky bugger to fuck off," Rita said.

"You've just got such a gift with words." I smiled.

"I hear you're on your own again," she continued, changing the subject.

"Blimey," I said. "Would it be easier for everyone if I put a regular update of my personal life on the noticeboard in the community center?"

"No need." She laughed. "Every bugger knows it all anyway."

"But how?" I asked in amazement.

"Easy. My sister-in-law's cousin works at the airport. She told everyone she saw you having a pash with some fancy bird about to catch a flight to Paris a few months ago. You've been a right pain in the arse ever since, and two and two make four."

"Wow!" I said. "You were paying attention at school after all."

"Anyway," she continued, ignoring my interjection, "since whoever it is has obviously pissed off on you, what are you doing about it? Anyone on the horizon?" she asked.

"Too busy," I replied.

"Too busy to have a bit of company? So who are you? St. Francis of fucking Assisi? Anyway, since everyone knows you're on your own again," she continued before I could answer, "I'll bet you're getting plenty of offers."

"No, never," I said after the slightest of pauses.

"Bullshit." She narrowed her eyes and looked at me.

"Well," I said, borrowing from Gilbert and Sullivan, "hardly ever."

Community interest in finding me a mate completely evaporated when Helen arrived on the scene. Word had obviously gotten around that Helen was now on the other side of the world, however. I had recently started being invited to dinner by one or two of the local single ladies, and another of my regulars had answered her front door topless when I called in response to her request for a house call. Apart from Liz, however, there was nothing that I hadn't been able to handle.

It was at about this time that Gabrielle was born. After the failure of their first marriages, Tom and Liz, who had met at the football club dance, surprised everyone by deciding to tie the knot after knowing one another for only a few weeks. They then moved into Tom's tiny cottage up near the trotting track and were joined there by the six offspring they had jointly accumulated from previous relationships.

Everyone who knew Tom shook their heads at his choice. Liz was not the community's favorite person and had the reputation of being sharp with her tongue and of never letting the truth stand in the way of a good story. She had spread some horrid rumors when Beck had fallen ill some years before and had, more recently, been the center of gossip concerning the sexuality of one of the local pastors.

For a while, however, the situation appeared to work well. Then Tayla, Tom's oldest, unexpectedly left and went to live in Queensland with an auntie. Not much was heard of her for a while until one evening when she calmly phoned her father and informed him that not only was he now a grandpa, but also that Liz was now a grandma.

It seems that if you blend two families of teenagers into a very small house, eventually nature will poke its head out from under the bedclothes.

Unfortunately, Gabrielle's arrival was not seen in the same blessed light that bathes many such events. On the contrary, her arrival signaled an outbreak of hostilities that eventually lead to the breakup of the family. Not only did Tom and Liz accuse one another of failing to adequately supervise and control their respective offspring, but the water became further muddied when a row broke out between Sam and Jacob, Liz's older two boys, who both laid claims to fatherhood.

Beth decided that, probably wisely given the circumstances, it would be best for her to stay in Queensland and keep Gabrielle all to herself. Tom seemed to accept Beth's decision reasonably well, but Liz, with no network of friends to fall back on, took it hard indeed.

These days, there are plenty of counselors to help in situations such as this, but there weren't back then. There wasn't a psychologist within fifty kilometers of Dixon's Bridge, and if any help was to be offered, then it had to be me.

It is unfortunate, therefore, that at least in this regard, my training helped me not one jot. I went through medical school in the days when it was considered appropriate that the only advice a doctor ever needed to give a patient with an emotional problem was to pull their socks up, keep a stiff upper lip, straighten their shoulders, pull themselves together, stand up tall, get a grip on themselves, and behave like a man. Whatever skill I had in this area was simply what I had picked up along the way.

Shortly after she and Tom parted company, Liz came to me looking for help.

"I don't know why you've taken that woman on," Heather said in that prim and proper way of hers when she heard that I'd agreed to help. "You should be going home at the end of the day and resting, not staying behind to help that troublemaker. You're barely coping with your own problems at the moment, let alone sorting out other people's."

"Thank you, Mother Hen," I replied, "but I'll be fine."

Despite Heather's forebodings, the first couple of sessions with Liz went well, and she seemed to make good progress.

"Told you," I said to Heather knowingly.

"You mark my words," Heather said as she wagged her finger at me.

There soon came a point, however, at which Liz stopped making any further progress and started saying that I was just taking Tom's side and not being there for her. I began to feel out of my depth and offered to refer her to see a specialist in Melbourne.

"I see," she replied angrily, "so now *you* want to dump me as well, don't you?"

"No, no, not at all," I hastily said, and against my better judgment, I offered her some more of my own time instead.

Our next meeting was at the end of a particularly busy day, and I was dog-tired. Liz spent most of the session weeping, and I tried my best to be supportive. It is not pleasant seeing anybody upset, and Liz's continuing distress over the matter of her granddaughter also touched a personal chord deep inside me. Toward the end of the session, as Liz sat sobbing inconsolably, in silent sympathy, I put my hand on hers.

In the kaleidoscope of events that form my working days, it escaped my notice that Liz cancelled her next appointment. I did notice that something was afoot, however, a few days later when Heather and Meaghan asked if they could see me together at the end of work.

"You both look very serious," I said lightheartedly.

"Yes," they said without smiling, "we are."

"Oh," I replied, "then perhaps I'd better sit down."

"I'm afraid we have some bad news," they said, and then went on to tell me that Liz was going around the neighborhood telling anyone who wanted to listen that I'd betrayed her trust and ruined her life.

I was stunned. "But what on earth is she talking about?" I asked in horror.

"She's saying that you deliberately got her on her own in the surgery the other evening and then made a pass at her," they said.

"But that's ridiculous," I exploded.

"Of course it is," they said, "but we thought you'd better know anyway."

"Yes, thank you," I said and spent the entire evening feeling sick in the stomach, and then having yet another appallingly restless night. Nel came in at some stage, got up on the bed, and lay down beside me.

"I thought Liz didn't have any friends," I said to Heather the next morning.

"Aye," she said, "but there are always those who'll listen to rubbish."

My first reaction was to simply ignore the whole thing and wait for the storm to pass. I phoned both my insurance company and Felix for advice, and they both advised me much the same.

Unfortunately, the plan failed in three important respects. The first was that the storm didn't pass. The second was that patients kept asking me confidentially if I'd heard what was going around. The third was that, rather than fade with time, the story got bigger. Within a week or so, there was even a rumor that I was about to be struck off.

I started getting tummy pains whenever I ate. I developed a tremor in my fingers, and whatever slight ability to sleep I still possessed flew right out of the window.

My imagination went into overdrive, and my throat went all tight when I received a letter from the medical board in the mail. The letter sat unopened on my desk for two days until Meaghan accidentally did the honors when she saw it still sitting there.

"The bill for your registration," she said as she opened it and, when I gave an audible sigh of relief, asked, "Why? What on earth did you think it was?"

▪ ▪ ▪

"So how are you traveling?" Rita asked me a day or so later on a visit to the surgery with yet another of her brood.

"Fine, just fine," I said flatly. "Why?"

"Because you not only look fucking awful, but you also sound fucking awful," she said.

"Well," I said. "I don't know if you've heard but—"

"You're the one who's always saying that what other people say or think of you is none of your fucking business," she interrupted.

"Well, yes, I know, but—" I started to explain, but Rita cut across me again. "I wouldn't give that woman, and you know who I'm talking about, the steam off my shit," she said. "And just remember, opinions are no different from arseholes anyway," she continued. "Every bugger has one. Now come and have some lunch with me again and talk about something else for a fucking change."

And then, thankfully, just a few days later, the gossip all stopped just as quickly as it had started.

"Are you alright?" Rob asked when I went around to have tea with Heather and him a few days later. "Because you look dreadful."

"Why does everyone keep saying that? I'm fine," I said. "I don't know what you're all going on about."

"Because…" Rob started to say and then stopped.

"Anyway," I said, "I'm sure things will get better now that all the recent nonsense seems to have blown over."

"Yes, indeed," said Rob, and something about the tone of his voice made me look at him.

"Why do you say it like that?" I asked.

"Well, Doc," he added quietly, "what I mean is, you've got Rita to thank for that, of course, haven't you."

I looked at him in amazement. "What on earth are you talking about?" I asked.

Rob looked quite startled. "You don't know?" he asked. "I thought everyone did."

"Know what?" I asked.

"Well, when things were getting more than a little ridiculous," he said, "and you were going down the gurgler, Rita went around and saw her."

"Liz, you mean?" I asked in amazement.

"Of course I mean Liz," he said.

"And what happened?" I asked.

"Apparently," Rob said, "Rita told Liz that if she didn't shut her mouth immediately, she'd break both her arms. I understand that Liz said she could bloody well do and say what she liked, and then Rita replied that if she did, then she'd break both her legs as well. At least that's what I've heard," Rob said and took a sip of his whisky.

"Wow!" I said and took a sip of my whisky too.

"Yes, I'm sorry I missed it," Rob said, "especially as I understand that there was a fair bit of pushing and shoving involved."

I drove home that night a thoughtful person indeed. Nel got up and stretched as I came in.

"Imagine someone who, without even being asked to, puts themselves on the line to save someone else's bacon," I said to her as I got her dinner ready.

"Mais les chiens toujours faire que,"[18] Chanel looked up at me and said.

▪ ▪ ▪

"I believe I owe you a rather big 'thank you,'" I said to Rita the next time I saw her.

"What for?" she replied evasively.

"You know jolly well what for," I said.

"Some years ago, there was a story going around about *me*," she said, "so I know how much it hurts. You can say all that 'what other people think about me' shit until your blue in the face, but it *still* hurts. Anyway," she added quietly, "that's what you do for people you love," and she enfolded me in her capacious embrace.

"As I was saying," I said when I eventually managed to disentangle myself, "thank you very, very much."

Then a thought occurred to me. "But how did other people know that Liz's story was rubbish."

"Oh, that's easy," she said. "I've been going around telling everyone you couldn't possibly be wanting an affair with Liz because you're already having one with me. Now just get your arse over to my place tonight, and we'll try getting some food into you again. You're looking more and more like a fucking stick insect."

---

18. But dogs always do that.

RECIPES FOR DISASTER

Piggy Tonight

1 pork fillet
1 bottle satay sauce

1. Slice pork and fry.
2. Cover with sauce.

13

ROXY

I was aware that one of the properties across the creek from Woongarra had been on the market for some time, but since I hardly knew the people who lived there, I hadn't taken much interest in the proceedings. What alerted me to the fact that someone new had finally moved in was the sound of gunfire early one Sunday morning, which lasted throughout the whole of breakfast time.

When it eventually stopped, and since I hadn't heard any screams or sirens, I decided to go and visit my new neighbors and say "hello" with a cup of sugar.

I finished my toast, put down the Dawkins I was reading, and hopped in the pickup. Although my place and the new neighbors' property shake hands across the creek, it is a fair way by road from one front gate to the other, and it took me a few minutes to get there.

When I reached my destination, I drove up the driveway to the house and parked next to a red-and-white F250. As I got out of my vehicle, I was taken captive by four small girls, with feathers in their hair, who sprang out of the bushes.

"You are our prisoner," said the tallest one fiercely.

"I can see that," I replied. "My name is Paul, and my rank is neighbor. Who are you?"

"We have no names in your language," she replied. "We are aliens from another planet."

"Ooh!" I said, taking a step back, "Well, since I'm your prisoner, you had better take me to your lizard."

"Lizard?"

"Leader."

"Follow me," she said as she frowned at me severely and led the way indoors.

When I got inside, it took a few seconds for my eyes to adjust to the dark. Then, as my vision returned, I found, to my complete and utter amazement, that I was in the presence of God. He was sitting amid a sea of half-emptied packing cases and having a beer.

I am not sure how everyone else is with all the God stuff, and I am not even really sure how I am with it myself, but something seems to make the universe stick together, and I guess that it might as well be called God as anything else.

From time to time, I wonder what the universe-sticking-together mechanism might look like if he, she, or it ever chose to walk, crawl, or float among us. Being a traditionalist at heart, I picture a male humanoid. He would be large and fierce, but there would also be a dark and subtle wisdom about his eyes. He would have his head shaved to accentuate his fierceness and wear large gold earrings and a chain to demonstrate his strength. Yet while you might start wondering where the nearest exit was as soon as you caught sight of him, at the same time you would instinctively know that he was gentle and kind.

And, almost unbelievably, here he was. He flicked off the TV, butted his cigarette into his stubby, stood up, narrowly banging his head on the ceiling, and shook my hand with a paw that looked as if it might have once belonged to a bear.

"Andrew," he rumbled like a Norse deity.

"Paul," I replied, trying to sound more baritone than tenor.

"He called you a lizard," said one of the smaller aliens.

Andrew looked down at them and then shook his head as if to clear it. "What?" he said.

"He called you a—"

"Go on. Bugger off, the lot of you," he said to the girls. "Can't you see I've got company?"

The girls defied him for just a moment, then Andrew took a half step forward and they scattered like chaff before the wind. When the last patter of footsteps had died away, he opened the fridge, got out two beers, and handed me one.

"Get yourself outside of that," he said and sat down again.

"So, four girls," I said after moving some boxes and finding a half-carved wooden rhinoceros to sit on.

"Nope," he replied. "Five. There's also Roxy, the oldest, but she lives in Sydney. Won't have a bar of me, thanks to what her mum puts in her ear about me. Haven't seen her in years."

"That's a pity," I replied.

"So how come she lets you see the others?" I asked.

"Because, my friend," he replied with a sly smile as he leaned forward, "they are not all sprung from the same stock. Five different girls, five different mothers."

"Wow!" I said. "Now that *is* impressive."

"None of them live with me, thank God," he hastened to add. "I guess I kept trying for Tom Tiddle-oh, but he just never happened, and I've given up on him now. So every second weekend, wherever I am, the place fills up with girls."

"And the gunfire?" I asked.

"Ah," he said, "you heard that?"

And it seemed that I had better get used to it. Apparently, Andrew's early mornings were driven, in equal parts, by the dual needs of keeping cockatoos off his newly established vegetable garden and of killing something before breakfast. Apparently, it gave him an appetite.

"So that would account for the feathers." I nodded to myself in sudden understanding.

We chatted for a while, exchanged neighborly details, pledged mutual help as required, finished the beers, and then went outside to be surrounded by aliens once more. As I got into the pickup, I saw the sugar container sitting on the passenger seat.

"You don't need any sugar, do you, by any chance?" I asked tentatively.

"As a matter of fact, I do," he rumbled unexpectedly. "I can't find it anywhere, and the girls made an awful fuss at breakfast," so I handed it over. "Well, see you later," he added and banged on the side of the pickup as I drove off, feeling no sense of confusion whatsoever.

▪ ▪ ▪

Many years before, and only shortly after my move across the globe, I had been invited to a get-to-know-the-neighbors barbeque a few houses down from where I had bought a house in Melbourne. It had been a very pleasant afternoon, and I had congratulated myself on what a nice group of people my new neighbors all seemed to be. As I was leaving, several of my newly made friends had waved to me and called out the same thing, "See you later."

I got home wondering if I had inadvertently invited anyone back for drinks. I couldn't remember doing so, but in view of the parting words, I put some wine in the fridge, got out the biscuits and dip, tidied up the sitting room, and sat back waiting for my guests to arrive.

I continued to wait patiently for several hours. I eventually finished off the wine and nibbles myself, but even as midnight came and went, I hung in there. It wasn't until the early hours that a rather puzzled Englishman climbed the stairs and hit the hay.

These days, of course, I am much better at the local patois and fully understand that "see you later" doesn't mean that anyone is going to see anyone else later at all.

I also well remember turning up to my first Christmas function with a plate. I had thought it an odd request on the part of my hostess but had simply assumed that she was a bit short of crockery.

▪ ▪ ▪

It was always easy to tell from the sound of gunfire whether Andrew was at home or not. Occasionally, over the following months, whenever I heard a fusillade, I would give him a call, and we would get together for a beer and a bite to eat. Sometimes, the get-together was at my place, sometimes it was at his, and occasionally, when the girls were visiting and the barometer was showing fair, it was down on the banks of the creek that divided our properties.

From the very beginning, I enjoyed the company of this "man mountain" and continue to do so to the present day. In fact, apart from just two occasions, our times together have only ever been filled with laughter and man-talk, and trying to get the girls to leave us alone, for God's sake.

Owing to my lack of expertise in the kitchen, Andrew has been the cook on almost every occasion. He does not have an extensive repertoire, but he does have a formula, and he sticks to it like glue. Which means, of course, that whatever he cooks, it always tastes the same.

"Why do you always put in so many onions?" I once asked.

"Because I love 'em," he replied with a burp, and that has always been that.

Most times Andrew hits the culinary jackpot, but one evening, he produced a complete fizzer. He called it a casserole, but it was like trying to eat bricks. We both stolidly and silently chewed our way through the masonry for a while but eventually reached a point of exhaustion and gave it all to Seth, Andrew's old pig dog, and Nel, who both loved it.

"What on earth was that?" I asked with a grimace as I washed away the taste with some beer. "I've always been led to believe that you shouldn't use roadkill as an ingredient," I added.

Andrew was a bit offended. "No, no, you're mistaken," he hastened to reassure me. "That was off the property. It just needed a little more marinating."

"Off the property?" I exclaimed.

"Yes," he replied, "I shot it a few days ago. A possum. You've had possum here many times here before," he continued. "Just must have been an old one or something."

■ ■ ■

Between our meals together and my seeing the girls from time to time at the surgery, Andrew and I got to see quite a bit of one another. He also started coming over and helping out at with jobs at Woongarra. I was often stuck in the surgery, unable to get things done, and he was always keen for a bit of cash.

Andrew should really be called Jack, of course, for there isn't anything he cannot turn his hand to. When he isn't clearing a fallen tree on Woongarra, he is fixing a friend's car, installing a neighbor's security system, relocating a weatherboard, welding something up, or smoking someone's fish for them. For a while he even sold life insurance. But for all that, to this day I still don't really know how he makes ends meet.

One evening, when the girls weren't there and we'd had a couple of beers, I asked him about Roxy.

"I really miss her," he said. "I love all the others, of course, but she's my firstborn. She's coming up for sixteen in a month or so, and it would be nice to see her for her birthday."

"Well, why don't you send her a card and invite her over then," I suggested.

"Yes," he replied as he drained his stubby, "why don't I?"

■ ■ ■

A week or so later, unable to sleep yet again, and making myself a cup of tea in the early hours of the morning, I heard gunfire from across the creek. Andrew usually placed a strict curfew on his shooting, so I gave him a call.

"Come on round," he said, "and see what I've caught."

From time to time, Andrew confided in me, when he got a bit lonely of an evening, he would phone round whichever of his ex-wives he was speaking to at the time and see if anyone was interested in coming over for a bit of slap and tickle. Apparently, somebody always was, and on the night in question, he had been joined by Jane. She and Andrew had dined together and then retired early, presumably to see what needed slapping and also what might need tickling, after which they fell into a deep relaxing sleep.

During the small hours, however, Jane's slumbers were interrupted by the noise of what she thought was Andrew rummaging around the house looking for something. She had then turned over, only to find that he was still sound asleep in bed next to her.

"I think there's someone in the house," she whispered in his ear as she shook his shoulder.

Andrew not only woke immediately, but also took Jane's suggestion to heart for, at the very moment he opened his eyes, he saw two darkened silhouettes flit across the end of the bedroom.

Now in a situation such as this, I am not sure what anyone else would do, but I feel that I could easily have a strong inclination to pull as many bedclothes over my head as possible and stay quietly huddled underneath them until whoever it was had gone home. On a brave day, I might quietly call out "Excuse me!" and hope not to be hit on the head by a piece of four by two.

Andrew, on the other hand, acted very differently. Without a moment's hesitation, he grabbed the gun from under the bed, the ammunition from under his pillow, and fitted the latter into the former. He then charged naked through the house, making a citizen's arrest of the two South Sea Islanders he caught in the kitchen. He then made them lie face down on the front lawn and tethered their hands behind their backs with cable ties. He then fired a few shots into the night to let everyone know he meant business, just in case they hadn't already caught on, got dressed, and called the police.

When the police finally arrived, some half an hour after I did, they went berserk. Far from being pleased at being presented with villains caught red-handed, and trussed up ready for transport, the boys in blue saw the episode in a very different light altogether. They carried on about unlawful arrest, insisted that the lads on the lawn be released immediately, and got stuck into Andrew for having a gun under his bed.

"What the hell did you expect me to do?" he exploded.

"Stay within the law," one of them said, thrusting his face up at Andrew, and just for one glorious moment, I thought Andrew was going to clock him one.

The islanders, relieved to be standing once more, and rubbing life back into their wrists, were frisked by the police. They had no contraband on them, of course, since Andrew had already retrieved all his belongings so, to our amazement, they were simply given a warning and escorted off the property. Andrew, on the other hand, was roundly ticked off for quite some time and informed that he might well be hearing more about the matter at a later date.

The whole episode seemed to fly in the face of every concept I have ever held about crime and justice. Having a steadying nip with Jane and Andrew after the police finally departed, however, it was obvious that it was only Jane and I who were frothing with indignation. Andrew, man of the moment, appeared surprisingly calm about the whole thing.

"You seem surprisingly calm about it all," we observed.

"Yes, well." He chuckled quietly. "It did occur to me that it might turn out this way, especially when I took all my stuff back off them. So I borrowed a leaf out of your book," he said, looking at me slyly, "and decided to be neighborly."

"What do you mean?" I asked.

"Well, between getting dressed and phoning the police," Andrew smiled at us, "I filled up a cup with sugar, walked down the road to where the boys had parked their panel van in the shadow of some trees, and emptied it into their petrol tank."

▪ ▪ ▪

Just a few days after her birthday, Andrew unexpectedly got a call from Roxy in response to the card and the scarf that he'd sent. She said she was prepared to come down for a weekend, but only if the other girls were going to be there as well. Andrew was delighted and fixed a date with her right there and then. She was to fly down on the Saturday morning, and he would pick her up from the airport. He talked about little else over the next week or two and was clearly tickled pink.

The night before Roxy's visit, there was a spectacular storm, and it was still gusting and raining heavily on the morning of her much-anticipated arrival. Andrew checked that the flight was still scheduled, and then, leaving the girls at home to clear breakfast away and set up an extra bed, he headed off to pick her up.

Almost immediately, Andrew knew he was not going to be on time. Not only were there fallen limbs everywhere, but the road to the airport had flooded during the night and was impassable. Frustratingly, he had to double back and go the much longer way round through the hills. Even here, the going was slow. When Andrew finally reached the airport, he was almost an hour late.

Roxy's flight had long since landed, so he drove round to the pick-up area looking for her and eventually found her huddled in the corner of a bus shelter. She was cold, wet, and furious in the belief that her father had engineered her discomfiture deliberately.

Apparently, Andrew had to look twice to be sure it was Roxy for she had grown so tall. Without even glancing at her father, however, Roxy threw her sodden suitcase onto the back seat and got into the vehicle.

"Mum said she thought you'd pull some stupid stunt like this," she said spitefully and then turned and looked out of the side window.

"Hi, lovely to see you, Roxy," Andrew was going to say, but he glanced across at his daughter's angry profile, checked himself, and pulled away from the curb without saying a word.

By the time they reached the road that climbs up through the hills, the silence in the vehicle had taken on a life of its own, and they both seemed frozen within it. Andrew had started to speak several of times, but Roxy had not responded at all. It was not at all the start that Andrew had wanted, but he had no idea what to do about it.

There are a number of difficult corners on that road, and about three-quarters of the way up, there is a particularly awkward bend that tightens up as you enter it. At this point, the road also flattens out a little, and the rain had pooled there, forming a skating rink of wet bark and leaves.

A new limb had come down on this bend since Andrew had passed through shortly before on his way to the airport. Unsighted, he was almost upon it before he saw it and had to swerve at the last minute. Normally, Andrew is a perfectly safe driver, but on this occasion, perhaps focused more on the silence in the car than on the road, he got it all wrong. As he took evasive action, he lost control of the F250. It skidded sideways across the road, crashed down an embankment, and slammed sideways into a huge gum tree.

It was all over in just a few seconds. When the violence of the moment came to an end and when, apart from a persistent hissing from the radiator, everything became quiet again, Andrew laughed out loud with the knowledge that he had come through it all without so much as a scratch.

"Thank God," he shouted with relief to the sky and then turned to Roxy and touched her on the arm. "Are you okay too?" he asked. When she didn't reply, he leaned across and repeated more loudly, "Roxy, are you okay?"

But Roxy said nothing. She just lay back in her seat, staring at her father with unblinking eyes from an expressionless face. Then from the corner of her mouth, some blood slowly trickled down her chin.

"Oh, Christ!" yelled Andrew as he reached across to her. "Oh Christ, oh no! Oh Christ, oh no! Oh Christ!" he screamed as he pulled out his phone and frantically dialed for help.

▪ ▪ ▪

It was the ambulance service that passed the call on to me. Happening to be home, I flew out of the door and headed off into what was fortunately a lull in the storm. It was a frustrating journey, for although I wanted to get there as quickly as possible, the pickup kept sliding about, and I frequently had to slow down to what felt like a snail's pace.

And as I drove, I hoped as hard as I could that whatever was waiting up ahead might not be as bad as I feared. Just occasionally, things weren't as horrible as they sounded, I thought. I reflected that while I had been to many accidents where the number of human beings on the planet had decreased, there had also been many where that was not the case. There had even been one occasion when the number had gone up, when a passenger had given birth by the roadside.

And then I was there. I rounded a curve in the road and arrived at the scene at the same time as the ambulance, which was coming from the opposite direction. Andrew had pulled Roxy up the bank on to the roadside and was giving her mouth to mouth.

He was exhausted, so David, the ambulance officer, and I immediately took over. We worked on Roxy until our backs and arms ached and then we worked on her some more, but there was never even the slightest flicker of response. Eventually, we agreed that there was simply no point in going on, and we stopped pounding her poor little body. Neither of us moved. We just stayed where we were, kneeling either side of her, looking down at her in silence.

"What a beautiful girl," David said. "I have a daughter about her age," he said wistfully. "We don't get on too well, unfortunately," he added and then got up and went over to sit with Andrew.

"Poor Roxy," I said quietly as I continued to kneel by her side, and as I spoke, the skies opened up yet again and the rain poured down. "We never even met, and yet you are now a part of my life," I whispered to her, and a great wave of loss rose up and washed over me. My head sank on to my chest, and my mind filled up with the memories of all those who had gone before.

I have no idea how long I stayed by Roxy's side, but at some point, I became aware that David was calling out to me. "Are you okay?"

I suddenly realized that I was drenched and freezing cold.

I looked at the rain splashing on Roxy's beautiful, unlined face, and I reached down and closed her big blue eyes. I then wiped my face on the back of my wet sleeve, put my emotions back in their box, shut the lid, turned the key, stood up, and went over to speak to the police who had just arrived.

"Are you sure you're okay?" David asked again as I passed him.

"Yes, I'm fine, thanks," I replied.

Despite much encouragement, Andrew refused to go to hospital for a checkup, saying that he just wanted go home to his girls. So that when Roxy had been taken away in the ambulance, and the police had completed all that they needed to do, I put Andrew in my pickup and drove him home.

The girls, who had been so excited at the prospect of Roxy's visit, were devastated. I made tea and cordial for everyone and then stayed on as, little by little, the crying gradually settled.

"Did you get to say much to her?" I asked Andrew quietly when the time seemed right. "No," he replied simply with his head hung down. "When I first picked her up from the airport, we didn't say so much as two words to one another. But when it was obvious we were going to crash," he continued, looking up at me, "we reached out and held hands."

Then like a man waking from a dream, he got up and said, "I have a job to do," and he walked through to the sitting room where I heard him pick up the phone and dial.

"Diane, it's Andrew. No, don't put the phone down on me this time. There's something I have to tell you," I heard him say as I let myself out.

■ ■ ■

As I drove home, I was dreading spending the evening on my own, but I needn't have worried. With uncanny timing, Mark had dropped by for another visit and was waiting for me. We didn't say anything. We didn't need to. We just sat and had a drink together.

The rain was still pouring down when I went to close the curtains. As I did so, the pattern of the rain running down the outside of the windowpanes formed itself into the shape of Roxy's face, and I was able to hold back no longer. I turned, put my head on Mark's shoulder, and as he hugged me, wept as I hadn't wept for many a long year.

14

PAUL

When I woke up, although the morning was well underway, I didn't have the faintest idea where I was. I had a memory of having been visited several times during the night, and of people shining torches in my face, but that was all.

I got up and sat on the edge of the bed and tried, without success, to shake my head clear. A nurse came in and said she was pleased to see me awake at last, and would I like to come through for breakfast, but to be careful as the medication I'd been given the night before could have made me wobbly. I put on the dressing gown she handed me and looked around for the cord until she told me that there wasn't one.

Around the breakfast table sat eight or ten others. None of them looked up at me as I came in. They were all eating in silence, and they were all wearing exactly the same dressing gown that I was wearing. As I sat down, I looked round at my companions and wondered who on earth they were. I was obviously in a hospital, but I seemed to be *with* other patients, not looking after them.

After breakfast, I walked round the room a little and found a windowsill where I sat and looked out at the rain. I was asked several times by the nurses if I was all right, and though I still felt very confused, I nodded that I thought I was.

As the day wore on, my head gradually cleared. Late that afternoon, and without any warning, the fog suddenly lifted and I remembered everything in absolute clarity. I remembered the ride to the hospital in the ambulance, and I also remembered what had happened before.

These days, looking back, it is obvious to me that I'd been falling ill for some time, but then I guess hindsight is always like that. At the time, it hadn't seemed to me like that at all.

I knew that I was staying longer and longer at the surgery each day, but I put it down to conscientiousness. I knew that I had become irritable with Meaghan and Heather, but I put it down to them being difficult and uncooperative. I was aware that I was sleeping less and less, but all I said was, "There'll be plenty of time for sleeping in the next world."

"I don't know how you get so much done," people would say, and I took it as a compliment, and then shifted the goalposts again and drove myself even harder.

I didn't even see any problem when I lost so much weight that I had to cut new holes in my belt.

"I've always wanted to be slim," I said.

"Yes, but are you sure you're not overdoing it?" people would reply.

I look back at the passport photograph I had taken during that time, and seeing that haunted man who looks back at me with sunken eyes, I am puzzled as to how I could have missed that something was dreadfully wrong.

I am equally amazed that nobody else picked it up either, but that may not be true for, although I can't remember them doing so, many people have since said that they tried to warn me. Maybe they were simply wishing they had, but then again maybe they really did and I just wasn't well enough to hear them.

I have often gone over the events leading up to my hospital admission. I was desperately upset about Helen, of course, and her absence gnawed at my insides more with every passing week. It felt as if a part of me was missing. I was also overwhelmed by the workload after Felix left. The episode with Liz had certainly been horrible and the image of closing Roxy's eyes in the rain were with me every day, but in the end, it was Geoffrey who proved to be the final straw on the camel's back.

On my own, and with all the weekend and night work on top of the normal busy week, even I eventually came to see that I needed a break. Felix, bless his heart, came up from town to help out from time to time, but what I really needed was another permanent pair of hands in the practice.

"You look so tired," patients would say. "Why don't you get some help?"

"Why, do you know someone?" I would reply hopefully.

"No, but what about a locum?"

"Well, I suppose I could," I'd reply half-heartedly, but I wasn't really that keen.

Felix and I had taken on a few locums over the years, but in all truth, they hadn't been particularly successful. There had been the one who had insisted on having a nana-nap between patients, causing him to run hours behind schedule. And there had been the one who had stopped everyone's contraception, seeing it as an abomination in the eyes of the Lord, and causing several unplanned additions to the community.

Despite my misgivings, however, Heather did eventually bully me into agreeing to take some time off. A replacement was duly organized from an agency, and I picked him up from the railway station on the Friday afternoon that I was due to go on leave. We had initially planned to have someone who had helped out satisfactorily in the practice some time before, but he had pulled out at the last minute on the excuse that his wife had gone into labor. Geoffrey was his stand-in.

Geoffrey seemed pleasant enough as I showed him around the farm and the surgery. I handed him my home visiting bag, showed him where all the keys lived, gave him my emergency torch, wished him well, and left for what even I saw as a well-earned break.

I was quite excited. Not only was I going to stay with some friends who lived next to a trout stream in New South Wales, but they also mentioned that they would like to introduce me to an acquaintance of theirs, a lady doctor who could well be interested in country practice.

The farm where my friends live is remote indeed. Getting there involves two plane rides and a long and bumpy journey in a four-wheel drive. I didn't arrive until late in the evening, but even so, dinner was still waiting for me.

"Sit down and relax," my hostess said as she poured some wine, and I did exactly that.

"This is chicken soup for the soul," I said after we had finished our meal and stretched out by the fire with the dogs.

But it wasn't to last because unfortunately things weren't going quite so well back home.

Shortly after I left, Geoffrey found my whiskey decanter and drank it dry. He then fell asleep on the living room couch, burning a large hole in the washed Chinese rug with the cigarette that slipped from his fingers as he drifted into unconsciousness.

It was probably the telephone call from Dymphna at Shangri-La that saved the house, and perhaps even the whole farm, from going up in flames. She had called to ask for help with one of the residents. Geoffrey was eventually awakened by the persistent ringing of the phone and, after lifting the receiver, asked whoever was on the other end of the line to hold on while he put out the fire.

"Did you say 'fire'?" Dymphna asked.

"No," he reassured her after a minute or two. "There's no fire now."

"Well, in that case, could you please come and see Betty," Dymphna continued. "I'm really worried about her breathing."

"Pardon?" he said.

"Could you come and see a patient at the old people's home," Dymphna repeated a little slower and louder. "I am worried about her breathing."

"Worried about her what?" Geoffrey said.

"Her breathing," Dymphna shouted in exasperation.

"Her bleeding?" he said.

"Oh god," said Dymphna.

It was some time before effective communication took place, but eventually, Dymphna got her message across and Geoffrey agreed to attend.

As I don't have a CCTV in my house, I will never be completely certain as to what happened over the next few hours. It does appear, however, that after speaking to Dymphna, Geoffrey found a second bottle of scotch in the pantry and drank that as well.

What I do know for a fact is that at two o'clock the following morning, Geoffrey drove my pickup into the parking bollard at the front of Shangri-La, crawled through the front door on his hands and knees, fell over a chair in the reception area, and then vomited into a wastepaper basket.

Dymphna, who had stayed on at the end of the shift because of her concerns about Betty, together with Ingrid who was doing the overnight duty, somehow managed between them to get Geoffrey into a chair in the nurses' room. They poured copious quantities of black coffee down his throat and also, since he had peed himself, cleaned him up as best they could. After a while, he was able to stand.

"I have come to shee a payshunt," he announced.

"Mush shee payshunt," he insisted. "Thash what I'm here for," so one on either side, Dymphna and Ingrid reluctantly guided Geoffrey down the hallway. When they reached Betty's room, Geoffrey pulled down the bed sheet and leaned forward over her, swaying gently back and forth. After a while, he slowly straightened up and turned to Dymphna.

"Doesh she always look ash bad ash zhish?" he asked.

"No, Doctor," Dymphna replied politely, "but then she has, after all, been dead now for just over two hours."

"I think it is now time," Dymphna continued, "for you to go back to wherever you came from. I will get Heather to organize a driver for you, and we will let Dr. Carter know what has happened."

Dymphna drove Geoffrey back to the surgery and left him in my consulting room. An angry Heather, awoken from her sleep, arrived shortly after to let Geoffrey know that she had organized a driver to take him back to town. Any of his stuff at the farm, she had decided, could be sent on later.

In her temper, Heather stormed into my room, to speak to Geoffrey, without knocking. Although she had intended letting Geoffrey know exactly what she thought of his performance, as she threw the door open, she stood motionless in shocked silence. The ampoules from my medical bag were scattered all across my desk, and Geoffrey was sitting in my chair with a syringe full of narcotic jammed into his left thigh.

"Oh my god," shrieked Heather when she found her voice again, and rest of the story can be read in the minutes of the medical board meetings.

▪ ▪ ▪

"I am so sorry we had to call you back," Heather said to me the next day when she picked me up from the airport.

"Not nearly as much as I am," I replied tiredly.

"Anyway, tell me, what was the lady doctor like?" she asked on the way back.

"I have no idea," I said resignedly. "I never even got to meet her. I left before she arrived."

▪ ▪ ▪

It was shortly after having to return to the practice and stand in for my own locum that my brother started visiting me again.

"Hi, Mark!" I would say with a smile. "Back again?"

"Just thought I'd check in," he would reply. "Sorry to hear about Geoffrey."

"Yes, what a muck up that was," I would say, and then over a glass of whatever, we would chat on for ages about this and that.

"I really enjoy your visits," I would eventually say to him, "but I'm feeling a bit sleepy now."

"Well, in that case, I'll leave you to get some rest, and I'll come back another time." He would smile back at me.

Eventually, Mark started visiting almost every day. It was usually of an evening, but occasionally he would also come when I was out working on the farm. He never stayed very long, but it was always nice to see him.

"Just popping by to see how you are traveling," he would say.

"How nice," I would reply. "Please come again."

I never told anyone else about him. It was not that I deliberately kept him a secret, but simply more that it never even crossed my mind to do so.

"So how are you really going?" he asked me one night.

"In all truth," I confessed with a sigh, "not as well as I would like."

"I didn't think so," he replied.

"I feel so agitated about everything all the time," I said.

"Like what?" he asked gently.

"Like, I'm no good at my job," I replied. "Like, I'm no good at even running my own life. I mean, what do they all think about me?"

"What other people think—" he started to say.

"Yeah, yeah, yeah," I interrupted him. "I know all that, but it still doesn't stop me worrying about it."

"Does the dog help?" he asked.

"Which dog? Oh, you mean Nel," I replied. "A bit, I suppose. She's certainly better than she was at the start."

"Good," he said brightly. "Always think of the positives."

And then one day, I started having other visitors as well. Visitors who I didn't know. Unpleasant visitors.

"Call yourself a healer?" they would sneer.

"You're just a filthy sleaze," they would shout at me.

And over the weeks that followed, the new visitors became ever more numerous, and their voices became ever louder. Eventually, there were whole courtrooms of them screaming "guilty" and "failure" both day and night. And somewhere in amongst all that, Mark stopped calling.

Looking back, I have no idea how I functioned during that time, but I did. I kept up my normal routine and even managed a cheerful appearance some of the time, but an invisible cloak of loneliness had settled over me.

"Are you okay?" patients would say when, halfway through a consultation, I would drift off into my own secret screaming world.

"Sorry," I would say as I forced myself back into the present. "Yes, of course."

"Are you sure you're okay?" they would persist as they looked at me closely. Even now, I can't explain why I never told anyone else what was going on. I just didn't.

Then at home one night and watching the evening news, I saw a bulletin about a young girl who'd been killed in a car crash. The report showed pictures of an F250 wrapped around a tree.

It was nothing to do with anything I had been involved in, of course, but I sat paralyzed by the images on the screen and, for a moment, even thought that the pictures were somehow those of Roxy's crash. I eventually shook myself out of it, but that night, the voices screamed incompetence and abuse more loudly than they had ever done before.

At around two o'clock the next morning, the voices reached such a crescendo that my only thought was one of escape. Calmly and methodically, I went outside. I gathered together everything that I needed and put it all at the back of the pickup. I then drove down to a clearing in the bush down by the creek on the edge of the property and parked in among the trees. I taped one end of a garden hose to the exhaust and poked the other end through the back window. I then turned on the ignition, closed my eyes, sat back, and prayed for relief.

▪ ▪ ▪

I spent many days sitting on that windowsill in the hospital dayroom, and little by little, I started to recover. I wasn't at all cross at finding myself alive, as I'd heard others say in similar circumstances, for ending it all had never been my motive. All I'd ever wanted was for the screaming to stop.

▪ ▪ ▪

Many years before, when my first marriage unfolded, and knowing that I needed to do something extremely different to take my mind off things, I had joined an expedition to Everest.

"Isn't that a bit dangerous?" everyone had asked.

"Who cares," I had answered carelessly.

But in the middle of a stormy night, three parts of the way up Everest, I realized that I did care, that I really did want to continue with life. One night, huddled up with other expedition members against the extreme cold, in a small tent that threatened to disappear off into the blizzard at any moment, I realized I couldn't breathe. I tried sitting up, then kneeling, but it made no difference. Realizing that my lungs were filling up with water from the altitude, I woke up my Sherpa. I thought I was going to die that night as we left the relative safety of the tent and climbed back down the mountain through the storm. When, many hours later we finally made it down, in one piece, to the shelter of the valley below, I was overjoyed at still being alive.

■ ■ ■

And day by day, as I sat looking out at the hospital grounds, my medication weaved its miraculous modern magic. The screaming gradually faded away, and I was left with a silence that I realized I couldn't remember enjoying for a very long time.

And in that silence, I thought over all that had happened. I also found myself missing my visits from Mark, for I had enjoyed them. He was just ten minutes younger than me. We had been inseparable and had always known instinctively what the other one was thinking. We had spent our days together, making up games, riding our bikes, or exploring the woods at the back of our house.

Then one day while we were making something or other in the shed, Mark's legs had suddenly swelled up. There was no one home, and I hadn't known what to do. I eventually managed to get help from a neighbor, and that very same day Mark was taken to the hospital, and I never saw him again. I didn't even get to go to the funeral.

"Which just goes to show you how much things have changed," said the nurse who was sitting talking to me. "Do you think that's why you became a doctor?"

"Could be," I answered. "I've never thought of that before."

"I lost my whole family that day," I continued. "My poor parents were overwhelmed with their own grief, and I never had another birthday," I added after a long pause. "They could just never face that date again. Not that I'm complaining," I added quickly. "Everyone was really nice to me. I don't even know why I'm talking about all this old stuff."

"Perhaps because you need to," she continued. "Anyway, you look a bit better for it. Remember to always think of the positives," she added.

"That's what Mark says," I said.

"Used to say or still says?" the nurse said with a wry smile as she looked at me sideways.

"Used to say, of course," I said and winked at her.

And for no particular reason, as I sat and watched the world go by outside my windowpane, I thought of the chemistry set that Mark and I had been given for the last birthday we had shared together.

I'm sure that today's chemistry sets are all very politically correct, but they weren't back then. When we opened the box and saw that the first two recipes were for cyanide and dynamite, we could hardly believe our luck.

Making the cyanide was surprisingly easy. It was the field testing that proved difficult until a friend of ours offered his mother's cat as a test case. Frisky was extremely old and blind, could hardly walk anymore, and had become incontinent. She was being taken to the vet in the next few days anyway, he said.

We soaked some cat biscuits in our brew and put them in Frisky's bowl. The three of us then sat in a semicircle and watched silently as Frisky ate her last supper. For a few seconds, nothing happened, and our friend made derogatory comments about our scientific expertise.

Then, suddenly, and I understand for the first time in her life, Frisky lived up to her name. She catapulted herself up into the air, jumping from curtain to curtain around the room, only to fall lifeless on her bed a few seconds later. It was there that she was later found by our friend's mother, and praised for not only having passed away naturally but also for having done it with a smile on her face.

"What an awful story." The nurse wrinkled her nose when I told her.

"Perhaps it works better if you're a twelve-year-old boy," I said.

Unlike the cyanide, the dynamite didn't go unnoticed at all. Having made a test tube of the stuff, we decided, for reasons that must have seemed valid at the time, to test it out in our outside loo. We piled some bricks on top of our creation, lit a fuse, and retreated to what we saw as a safe distance. I think we were expecting a loud pop and a bit of smoke. What we got was a huge explosion that rattled the entire neighborhood. Our dynamite blew the entire structure to pieces. A brick flew past our heads, and what was left of the bowl finished up on the neighbor's roof.

"I still really miss Mark," I said to my mother when she came in to visit me.

"Me too," she said with a sigh.

▪ ▪ ▪

At everyone's insistence, I took an open-ended break after I was well enough to leave the hospital. I wasn't even certain if or when I would be well enough to practice again. But I didn't have to worry for this time Heather had found someone sensible to babysit the surgery.

"His name's not Geoffrey, is it?" I asked.

"How did you guess?" she replied and then, when I looked across at her, continued, "No, actually it's that nice man whose wife was having the baby." I drove up the coast, visiting various friends along the way and feeling ever stronger. After some weeks, I finished up in a caravan park at Brunswick Heads. I sat on the banks of the river on my first evening there, and sipping a cool beer, I looked up and saw the evening star.

I raised my drink to the darkening sky and thanked the star for my lucky escape.

"What on earth was I thinking about?" I murmured to it.

"You weren't thinking about anything," the star softly murmured back. "You were far too ill for thinking."

"Yes, you're probably right," I replied, and then a thought struck me. "You're not one of those voices, are you?" I asked.

"No," the star giggled. "I'm just a star."

"Good," I replied, "because just for a moment there, I was a bit worried. But tell me anyway, do you think I'll be okay to practice again?"

"If you make it happen," the star replied.

"Good," I said, "because I'm feeling heaps better, and I would certainly like to give it a go."

▪ ▪ ▪

Despite what I so often lectured to others, I spent most of the journey back home thinking about how people might react to my return. I imagined that just about everyone in the district would know what had happened.

Heather gave me dinner on my first night back. "You idiot!" she exclaimed as she smothered me with hugs and kisses. "Don't you dare even think of falling ill again without running it past me first."

"You're on," I said, and right there and then, I silently vowed to do whatever it took to ensure that I would never again wake up to find that my dressing gown cord had been taken away.

"I'm still a bit worried about facing everyone," I said.

"I can't think why," Rob replied. "You're no balmier than anyone else. I mean, half of them spend their Sunday mornings gathering together and then speaking to someone who's not there for a start off," he added and ducked as Heather threw a cushion at his head.

"Well, there is that," I said with a smile.

▪ ▪ ▪

"I heard you were back," Andrew said when he came across to my house the following night with a six-pack. "And since we're over at your place," he added, "why don't you do the cooking for a change?"

"Why not indeed," I replied and made us some chicken and corn.

"Jesus Christ," he said later, "you might be on the mend medically speaking, but you're still shithouse in the kitchen."

And then one evening, sitting on my own, gently toasting myself by the fire, Mark came and paid me one final visit.

"Are you meant to be here?" I asked him.

"It's a bit naughty, I suppose," he said, "but I just wanted to check that you really were okay now."

"That's very nice of you." I smiled at him. "Yes, I'm fine, thank you."

"Good," he said. "Well, that was all, so I'll be off then," he added as he waved goodbye, and I haven't seen hide nor hair of him since.

After Mark left, I got up and stretched. I stoked up the fire and then made myself a cup of tea. When I settled back down again, Nel came over and sat next to me.

"And as for you," I said, "there is, of course, one bit of very important unfinished business."

"Et qu'est-ce que c'est?"[19] she replied as she gazed into the flames.

"Well, just that I'd like to say a very big 'merci beaucoup' to you, Nel," I said. "A very, very big 'merci beaucoup' indeed from the very bottom of my heart," I repeated, and I reached down and stroked her woolly head.

"Ce n'etait rien,"[20] she replied demurely.

But it wasn't nothing, for the night that I drove the pickup down to the creek, she saved my life. Just a few seconds after turning on the ignition and closing my eyes, I was awakened by a thunderous scratching on the car door. I opened it to see what was going on and found Nel standing there, looking up at me. She

---

19. And what is that?
20. It was nothing.

must have followed me down to the creek to see what I was up to, and she put a paw on my leg.

I didn't know what to do. At first, I thought of pulling her into the car with me, but I couldn't do that so, for a moment, I just sat there trying to work out what to do next.

Eventually, I went to shoo her away, but the fresh air from the open door had made me dizzy, and as I reached down, I lost my balance. I cartwheeled out of the pickup and got stuck hanging out of the door with my foot wedged hard against the horn. Which is why, of course, Andrew came down to the creek a few minutes later to see what the fuss was all about.

RECIPES FOR DISASTER

Chicken and Corn

1 tin chicken soup
1 tin corn
1 stock cube

1. Empty soup and corn into a saucepan.
2. Add stock cube.
3. Boil.

15

NIGEL

One night, shortly after my return to work, I was called out to an emergency. I was just thinking of slipping between the sheets when Heather phoned and passed on an urgent message.

"Can someone come as soon as possible," Riz had pleaded with her. "Nigel can't breathe."

I asked Heather to organize an ambulance to meet me at the house, threw on the clothes I'd just taken off, and drove off at high speed into a cold and stormy night, splashing through the potholes that the recent bad weather had left in my driveway.

Nigel, who I had met briefly at a cricket match some time before, lived on the other side of Rushby at the foot of the Mullaways. Although the weather was filthy and I'd never been to the house before, the directions were good; and by disregarding a few road rules, I managed to break all existing time records in getting there. There are some requests for a house call that just cannot be put off, however tired one feels, and someone not being able to breathe is way up the list.

Riz had been spot-on in her diagnosis. Nigel certainly wasn't breathing well at all, and in the poor bedroom lighting, he looked a very nasty shade of blue. To my pleasant surprise, however, he had both pulse and blood pressure. A mask was popped over his face, and he was given oxygen by Ian, the ambulance officer who arrived at much the same time as I did.

"Well, he's breathing now," Ian said with relief, "so at least we don't have to put an airway in."

"I'd still like to call a chopper," I replied, "and I think we'll get a line up too."

"As long as they can make it in weather like this," Ian said, but despite the dreadful conditions, the air ambulance made a perfect landing in the lane beside the house just fifteen minutes later.

Nigel is a really big bloke, and his cottage is a really small one. There was just no way that we could get him out on a stretcher, so with a great deal of huffing and puffing, and assisted by the helicopter crew, we manhandled Nigel out of his bed and into the carport. Although there were plenty of hands on deck, it still took us quite a while. Carrying Nigel, together with assorted tubing and oxygen cylinders, round corners and up and down flights of steps that were never designed with this sort of thing in mind, was by no means easy. We repeatedly tripped over ourselves, bumped into furniture, and even managed to knock a picture off the wall.

The circus did eventually make it to the carport, however, and once Nigel's camouflaged Land Rover, with his regimental crest painted on the doors, had been backed out, it was a matter of simplicity to lay Nigel onto a stretcher and load him into the helicopter.

"Thank the Lord for that," I sighed to Ian as we completed the handover. "At least he's still alive."

We huddled in the scanty shelter of the carport waiting for the takeoff, but nothing happened. The rotors started to turn, but the wheels stayed on the ground.

For a moment, nothing seemed to be happening, and then the copilot jumped down and went around to the back of the machine.

"What's the problem?" we shouted out above the wind and the noise of the blades.

"Back door's not closing properly," he shouted back. "Ah, here's the problem. Never seen it before. Your bloke's too long to fit in, and his head's still poking out."

"What are you going to do?" we screamed.

"Give the door a bloody good push from the outside," he replied, and before either Ian or I could stop him, that is exactly what he did.

Even above the noise of the helicopter and the storm, we heard the door collide with Nigel's head, but even that didn't do the trick and the door flew open again.

The copilot was about to have another go at getting the door shut, but this time, we were too quick for him. Ian shot across and shouted, "Bend his legs!"

"What?" screamed the copilot.

"Bend his bloody legs!" Ian shouted again.

The copilot looked blankly at Ian for a second and then suddenly smiled, gave us a thumbs-up, and spoke on the intercom in his helmet. Inside the chopper, a crew member bent Nigel's knees up and pulled him into the machine.

The door with ease and the copilot was about to jump aboard when he turned and yelled, "Good thinking, boys. I'll remember that one."

Within seconds, the helicopter had risen up into the storm, and Ian and I went back into the house for a cup of tea with Riz before heading off to our respective homes.

"I wonder," Ian mused over his tea, "what sort of qualifications you need to crew one of those things. And by the way," he said, turning to me, "how are *you* feeling these days?"

"Much, much better thanks," I replied, "and many thanks for taking me down to the hospital that night."

■ ■ ■

A few days later, I arrived to do my first morning surgery back in Rushby after my break away. I usually liked to arrive early to get any paperwork organized, but I had accidentally slept in that morning and arrived with only a few minutes to spare.

I was hastily flicking through my correspondence when Meaghan popped her head round the door and gave me a cup of tea. She had a big smile on her face. Morning pleasantries were exchanged, and then I asked her what the grin was for.

"Because they're all here this morning," she said, "every last one of them. They've been hanging out for your return, and now you're back, they're all here. Together with a bonus," she added and disappeared back to her desk.

I put the paperwork to one side for later, swallowed the tea, which was several degrees too hot for comfort, and went into the waiting room to call in my first patient.

It was then that I realized what Meaghan had meant. The waiting room was packed. All my old favorites. All my old regulars. Every last one of them.

As I appeared, a small cheer went up and there was a chorus of "Glad to have you back, Doc" and "Hope you had a good break."

As I had driven back down the coast, I had been concerned about what sort of reception I would receive on my return, but I needn't have worried. I had also been concerned about how inquisitive people might be about my recent medical history, but just like Audrey's Harold before me, no one ever asked so much as a single personal question.

Normally, I would have given the assembled crowd a cheery hello and then asked who wanted to be the first cab off the rank. This time, however, I hardly even glanced at them for, standing to attention in the exact center of the room, was a giant of a man I didn't recognize.

By any stretch of the imagination, he was impressive. He must have stood almost seven feet tall and looked immaculate in his perfect military dress uniform. He wore mirror-polished patent leather shoes, and he carried a large and ornamental ceremonial sword. His shoulders, as far as I could tell, bore the insignia of some very high rank indeed.

"And who's first?" I said, looking around and sort of pretending not to have noticed him.

"I am, sah," he said in a laconic Alec Guinness–*Bridge over the River Kwai*-sey sort of voice that had just the faintest hint of a slur about it.

"Brigadier Carstairs," he continued, "British Army," and he shook me by the hand with a crush that left my knuckles stinging for ages. He then drew his sword out of its scabbard, touched it to his forehead, lowered it to the ground, then making his way through to my consulting room, using it as a walking stick.

"War wound?" I asked as we sat down.

"Gout," he said.

"Oh," I replied.

"Gout, old boy," Alec Guinness repeated as he breathed a little stale alcohol in my face, "is why I need to use a walking aid. Gawd knows why I'm afflicted. Must run in the family. Probably in the genes or whatever you call 'em. The good lady looks after my diet, and I never go through more than a couple of bottles of red a day, so it can't be that.

"But that's not why I'm here," he said, interrupting himself. "Just got out of hospital and came to say thank you. Was told you saved my life. I switched off the respiratory something or other, they said. Too much grog they said. Apparently, I should cut down, but there's not a chance in hell of that. So just came to say thank you for a jolly good show. Haven't been in a chopper since Northern Ireland."

"Ah," I said, eventually making the connection. I accepted his thanks graciously and let him know that Ian had also been part of the rescue team. After the exchange of a few more pleasantries, he got up to go. In the nick of time, I remembered to get my hand out of the way before it was crushed again, and I escorted him to the door saying how lovely it was to have met him again and how it had been my privilege to have been of help.

"Why don't you come around for curry one night with the memsahib and myself," he turned and said. "That is, if you like it hot."

"I certainly do," I replied. "That would be lovely," I added and promptly did nothing about it.

I saw Nigel several times more over the following weeks to check that his breathing was still functioning correctly. He was just fine, but he never made any changes to his lifestyle. On every occasion, he was always immaculately dressed and immaculately courteous. And on every occasion, I was just quick enough to avoid getting my hand crushed again.

Nigel would politely repeat the dinner invitation each time we met, and I would, just as politely, find an excuse. Since returning to work, I hadn't gone out much, preferring to stay in and have early nights. There came a time, however, when my refusals began to sound churlish, so I finally said yes, and a date was duly set.

"Is it okay if I bring my dog?" I asked, and apparently it was.

▪ ▪ ▪

The curry night at Nigel's was a fabulous evening. It was full of candlelight, silver service, and passing the port to whichever side is the correct one, in the tiny, falling-down cottage that Nigel and Riz call home. It was also an evening of G and S.

"Much better than any of that sloppy Italian muck," he said.

I raised an eyebrow and was about to reply but then I let it go and just hummed along with the Duke of Plaza-Toro.

Nigel, of course, was in full dress uniform that night while Riz looked sensational in a strapless ball gown. The conversation was sparkling, and the table constantly glittered as the flickering candlelight fell on the glassware and porcelain. In jeans and a jumper, I had initially felt a little underdressed for the occasion, but no one else seemed to mind, so I stopped worrying about it as well.

"Given to my great-great-great-grandfather for services rendered in the Americas," Nigel said as he put an ornate silver tureen of steaming curry on the table.

"Wow," I said, impressed, not just by the silverware but also by Nigel's faultless performance as both head chef and waiter, a task not made easier for him by ceilings so low that there was nowhere he could stand up straight. He spent the entire evening slightly bowed over, giving a wonderful *Alice's Adventures in Wonderland* feel to the whole proceedings.

The food was marvelous and certainly lived up to the promise of hotness. In answer to my questions, asked between drinking several gallons of water, Nigel told me that he'd learned the art of curry cooking as a lad in the Far East where his father had been a district commissioner for many years.

"I was born in Changi, as a matter of fact," he said proudly, "not long after the Japs were given the boot."

And as the meal progressed, inevitably we exchanged "coming out to Australia" stories. Nigel had come out a few years before me, but Riz had left Germany at about the same time that I had left England.

"Not a colonial amongst us." Nigel smiled as he looked round the table. "Apart from your dog of course," he added. "Although I guess she's French."

There was a brief lull in the conversation while we took some plates out to the kitchen, and then I asked Nigel how he liked living in Australia.

"Ghastly place," he replied. "Can't stand it really. As a country, it's only got two things going for it as far as I can see: the first is that they know how to lay willow on leather, and the second is that it's vastly preferable to anywhere else.

Sometime during the course of the evening, it started raining, and a whole cupboard full of assorted receptacles was brought out to cope with the leaks that suddenly appeared from everywhere. The noise of the water hitting the bowls was quite musical, and Nigel amused us by moving the various containers about until he had a surprisingly creditable version of *The Blue Danube*.

"Of course, if we had any spare cash," he said, "what we could do with is a hay shed."

"What do you mean?" I asked.

"It was in the paper recently," he replied. "Some fellow with a roof like ours found that, rather than repair all the leaks, it was cheaper to simply build a hay shed over the house."

"But I von't let him," Riz interjected, "because I like ze music."

Sipping on a glass of wine between courses, I gazed upon the wonderful array of decorations on Nigel's chest. My interest was increased by having recently admired some military medals that had been on display in the milk bar. They had belonged to a local war hero who, having returned home from the fray, had then lived out the rest of his life in his chook house.

I told Nigel that, whilst his chest was extremely impressive, I had no idea about such matters whatsoever and wouldn't be able to recognize a Victoria Cross from a St. John Ambulance badge.

"What are they all for?" I asked. "Especially those two?" I added, pointing to a matching pair.

"That, my dear boy," Nigel confided in me, pointing at the first of them, "is a military cross. And this," he continued, looking down at his own chest and pointing to the other, "is another military cross."

"Good Lord," I exclaimed.

"Two tours of duty in Northern Ireland, two military crosses," he said.

Even I know that military crosses don't grow on trees, and I was most impressed. "Can I ask how you got them?" I enquired.

"You certainly can," he said. "I got the first one for shooting somebody, and the second one for not shooting somebody else."

"Right," I replied, nodding my head in what I hoped showed a keen grasp of military protocol, and we recharged our glasses once more.

After we had recovered from the main course, Riz brought out the dessert. As she turned to put the bowls on the table, I realized that she had a tattoo on her shoulder blade. Frustratingly, I couldn't quite make out what it was, since there wasn't much of it showing, and each time she turned or moved, I had another quick peep.

Inevitably, Riz turned unexpectedly and caught me in the act. She blushed a little, laughed, and said, "Vud you like to zee him?"

It was now my turn to blush for being caught out, but I said yes anyway. Riz turned around and pulled the back of her dress a little way down. By the light of the candles, I could see the head and neck of a Doberman pinscher, with the name "Zu-Zu" inscribed in a scroll underneath. When Riz had readjusted her dress, she turned back to me with tears in her eyes.

"He vas a vunderful dog," she said with a break in her voice, "and ven he died I simply couldn't bear to be parted from him. Zo now he is viz me alvaze. You must feel zat about your beautiful dog too," she said and bent down and ruffled Nel's ears.

"I'm definitely getting there," I replied.

I've never had a tattoo, but for several days afterward, I toyed with the idea of having my previous dog, Hardy, emblazoned upon my person. I even asked Heather's opinion about the matter, but there is no way I could repeat her answer. In the end, I didn't go ahead with the plan and decided that I was happy just having a picture of him hanging in the kitchen.

At the end of the evening, I thanked them both for a lovely time, and then thanked them once again for sparing me any quizzing on my recent time away from the practice.

"Why, have you had some time off?" they replied with surprise. "Very wise," they continued before I could explain. "It does everyone good to occasionally get away and recharge the batteries."

"It wasn't quite like that," I said and was about to go into more detail, but then I stopped and simply let it drop. We made our final farewells, and as Nel and I got into the pickup, we promised that we would do it all again sometime.

Back home, I toyed with the idea of inviting them over for a meal at my place. I even practiced a tuna dish, but in the end, thinking of the gulf between their gold medal standards of cooking and entertaining, and how the pigeon evening had gone, I didn't have the courage.

I did continue to see Nigel on a regular basis in the surgery, however. Bit by bit he opened up about his medical past and revealed an entire encyclopedia of complex medical problems.

It took a lot of time and thought to work through all the issues with which he presented, and much was needed in the way of testing and specialist referrals. Bit by bit, however, every possible avenue of investigation was carefully ticked off the list, and I had all the reports and results in front of me. As far as everyone was concerned, Nigel was slap bang in the middle of every normal range that had ever been invented.

Then without warning or explanation, Nigel and Riz slipped off the radar and disappeared. When I first realized that they had gone, I popped up in the cottage to make sure that they were okay. It was locked up and everything seemed to be in order, so I simply left it at that.

Around four months later, and just as suddenly as they had left, there they were again, driving around town in the old Land Rover and acting as if they had simply been away for the afternoon. Apparently, they had been to the Isle of Man.

"Why on earth did you go there?" I asked

"Tax haven," Nigel answered in a hushed voice and tapped his nose.

"The trick," he confided in me, "is to always work to a scheme." He then gave me an impossibly complex account of his financial affairs, and not being savvy about such matters, I didn't have the faintest idea what he was talking about.

As the year came to an end, Nigel and Riz invited me over again for pre-Christmas nibbles. Having enjoyed myself so much on the previous occasion at their house, I accepted their invitation at the first time of offering.

I arrived pretty much on time, and the three of us arranged ourselves round a small table on the tiny disintegrating porch that clings precariously to the front of their house.

"I like ze decorations," Riz said, pointing at my flashing bow tie, which I had worn in the surgery that day at the insistence of Heather and Meaghan, who had both been wearing antlers.

I had felt a bit self-conscious when I first put it on but had then completely forgotten that I was wearing it. Which is why I had such a shock when, halfway through giving someone some really unpleasant news, I caught sight of my flashing reflection in my computer screen.

I reached up to my neck to try and discreetly turn the bow tie off, but the patient stopped me.

"Please leave it on," she said. "It's the only thing right now that's cheering me up."

The three of us nibbled and chatted and sipped. We were also careful not to lean on the table or let our chair's legs fall through any of the holes.

Halfway through proceedings, with Nigel and Riz both busy away from the table, I wandered into the front garden and looked back at the cottage. The entire place was in a dreadful state of repair. Every piece of timber was slightly out of true, and it was a long time since the outside of the house had seen any paint. The roof iron was all peeling away, the windows were rotting, and the exposed electrics looked positively dangerous.

"You can see why we love this place," Nigel said when he came back and saw me looking around.

"Yes, it's great, isn't it," I replied.

And nothing was ever done about any of it. The roof continued to peel, the windows continued to rot, the electrics flickered on and off the whole time, and every time it rained, Nigel played Strauss. I once suggested the need for a little maintenance, but they just looked at me in puzzlement and asked what I meant.

Riz brought a bottle of French champagne and three glasses back out of the house with her.

"To our wedding anniversary," they said in unison as they raised their glasses, and I joined in the celebration.

"Yes." Riz turned to me. "Von year today."

I guess it had just never occurred to me that they were newlyweds. I knew there was a son at university and had always assumed that he was the product of their union.

"No," Riz explained, "just von year today."

"So how did you meet?" I asked.

"I vas a tax accountant for a vile," Riz continued, "and Nigel came into ze office von day to talk about a scheme he had thought up."

"And was he in uniform?" I asked again.

"Vell, as a matter of fact, he vas," she replied with a blush and turned and smiled at him.

"What is it with women and uniforms?" I said. "Maybe I should get one."

We refilled our glasses and then asked one another what we were doing for Christmas. I was going to Melbourne to my mother's, and Nigel and Riz were staying at home to host Riz's parents.

"Sounds nice," I said. "Sounds like a lovely, quiet Christmas for all of us."

"Which is good," Nigel said, "because a few years ago it wasn't like that. A friend and his wife had come over to my place for Christmas lunch. At the end of the meal, he stood up and banged on the table for silence. I thought he was going to say how much he'd enjoyed the fare and to thank us for our hospitality, but he didn't. Instead, he said that he was now going to leave and that he was not leaving alone. My wife then stood up, and the two of them left together."

"Good Lord," I said.

"That was ten years ago," he continued, "and I haven't seen hide nor hair of them since. Don't think my son has either."

"And the rest of the party went well then?" I asked, and we all laughed.

■ ■ ■

Christmas came and went. Nigel was due to see me for a checkup in the New Year, but he didn't show up for the simple reason that he had run off with a BMW saleslady.

He had been talking for a long time about replacing the Land Rover and had gone down to Melbourne for a few days to look at what was on offer in the post-Christmas sales period. He was feeling pretty pleased with himself, for he had worked out some method whereby he could get his new car for free by simply putting it on the "army's account," as he explained, and getting it shipped out to Australia through the Channel Isles.

Apparently, a very nice BMW saleslady had taken him for a test ride and then, or so it seems, he had taken her out for one too. Clearly, lots of testing was needed, for he was away for some while. I never had the courage to ask him how it all panned out, but I do know that when he came back, he didn't have a BMW with him. Not once has Riz ever referred to the episode, however, and after his return, the two of them continued on as if nothing had ever occurred.

While he was away, and concerned as to how Riz was getting by on her own, I had taken it upon myself to investigate whether Nigel's army pension properly reflected the complexity of his medical problems. I'm not the best at finding my way through bureaucratic mazes, so I got Meaghan to give me a hand. Together we spent several hours of searching, but not only couldn't we find Nigel on any list, but we couldn't even find his regiment. "Shows you how good we are at this sort of thing," I said to her, and we shrugged our shoulders and admitted defeat.

One morning, shortly after Nigel's return, I was asked by Lesley, the practice nurse, if I could take a look at a patient who had just presented to the treatment room with some burns. I popped down the corridor a few minutes later to find Nigel, almost unrecognizable in dirty old clothes, lying face down on a couch with burns all over his bum.

Even from upside down, Nigel tried to give me one of his bone-crunching handshakes, but having by now had a good deal of practice at avoiding them, I simply busied myself with inspecting the damage. I discussed the treatment with Lesley and organized for Nigel to be reviewed by her on a daily basis for a while.

"How on earth did this happen?" I asked.

"Bloody motor mower," said Nigel in the clipped way he used when he was being official. "Just had it serviced. Twice round the back lawn. Damn thing exploded in flames. Got off in the nick of time. Insurance man's coming round later. Nearly lost me bollocks."

"Lawn?" I exploded. "No wonder your poor mower got overexcited. What you have behind the house waves in the breeze. It must be three feet high at least. There isn't the slightest lawn-like thing about it. What you needed was a combine harvester," I added.

Apparently, Nigel's neighbor had felt much the same. With summer in full swing, he had complained to the Shire about the fire hazard posed by Nigel's back garden. It was after a visit from some Shire officials that Nigel had dragged out his mower and brushed off the cobwebs.

Nigel's burns healed well over the next couple of weeks, but he was not a happy man when the insurance company chose to reject his claim for repairs and personal injury on the technicality that the lawn mower had never been designed or intended for agricultural work.

"They've picked on the wrong man this time," Nigel muttered darkly into the pillow on one of his visits to have his backside dressed. "Justice will be done, dear boy. Mark my words, justice *will* be done."

Eventually, the burns all healed, Nigel stopped coming for dressings, and the whole matter completely passed from my mind. Then one afternoon a few weeks later, I was interrupted by a telephone call from Melbourne.

"Can you take a call from a Mr. Stephenson of Mega Insurance?" Heather had asked.

"He's probably trying to flog me some life insurance, Heather. Just get rid of him for me please," I replied.

"I don't think so," Heather said. "He says he's the general manager and that it's urgent."

"Okay, okay, put him through, but I'll scrag you if he's selling life insurance. Good afternoon," I said with charm as the phone clicked over. "How can I help?"

"Dr. Carter? My name is Stephenson. We have a man here who is threatening my office staff with a sword. He is waving it about our front office and has poked it into the reception desk. He says he's a patient of yours and asked that I call you. Apparently, it's about a lawnmower. I was about to contact the police, but I thought that perhaps I should speak to you first."

I didn't need to ask who Stephenson's customer was. "So why don't you just settle his claim?" I asked

"That's exactly what I thought too," Stephenson replied to my complete surprise.

"He's harmless, you know," I added. "Maybe a touch eccentric, but there's no real chance of him hurting anyone. If you tell him you're paying up, I'm sure he'll put his sword away, so there's probably not much need to involve the police either, is there?"

"That's exactly what I thought too," Stephenson said again.

I couldn't believe my luck and was about to put the phone down. "He wasn't wearing a uniform, was he?" I asked.

"Well, yes, he's obviously a general or something."

"In which case, just make sure that none of your staff have fallen in love with him," I said, but I don't think he got it.

■ ■ ■

A few days later, I was on my way into the bank when I bumped into Nigel on his way out.

"They paid the claim," he said with a smile.

"Good," I replied.

"Showed them a bit of cold British steel," he continued. "They surrendered immediately."

"Very good," I replied, "but in future perhaps, you could keep your cold British steel in your cold British scabbard. And while I'm on the subject," I added, "how on earth did you get in and out of the Mega building carrying a rather large and pointy piece of metal without attracting the attention of security?"

"Stuck it down my trouser leg," he replied. "Got myself a disabled parking spot and limped."

Then something about the insignia on his shoulders caught my eye.

"The pips on your shoulders," I said with surprise. "There are more of them!"

There was a moment's hesitation, and the slightest flicker of discomfort crossed his face. In a fraction of a second, it had gone, and he smiled and said, "I've been promoted. The orders came through two days ago."

"How on earth could that be?" I asked in all innocence. "Don't you have to be on active service for that to...?" but there was no point in continuing, for he had already left.

RECIPES FOR DISASTER

Pasta con Tonno

¼ packet pasta
1 tin tuna

1. Boil pasta.
2. Mix in tuna.

16

PADRAIG

I had gotten on well with Father Padraig Aloysius O'Halloran from the very beginning. He is a tall man with an engaging personality and a great shock of hair that still shows traces of the red of his youth. He has a booming voice, perfect for sermons, and a laugh that rattles the windows. He also has a wicked sense of humor and the quick intellect you would expect of a man with a double first from Dublin University. He has lived in Australia a lot longer than I, but his delightful lilting brogue sounds as fresh as it must have done the day he stepped off the boat from Ireland.

When not attending to his flock, his passion is finches, which he breeds in the old aviary at the back of the rectory. The aviary had been there for as long as anyone could remember, and even when Father Padraig first arrived, I understand that it was more than beginning to show the signs of its age. Where the wire wasn't actually in holes, it was rusting through, and although Father Padraig had never lost any of his birds, he knew that it was only a matter of time before Mr. Rat or Mr. Fox came acalling and spoiled his fun.

Although not an experienced handyman, Padraig considered himself very much an all-rounder and decided to affect the repairs himself. He purchased the necessary materials from the hardware store, laid out his tools in a professional manner, rolled up his black sleeves, and set to. Unfortunately, with the very first swing of the hammer, he hit the wrong nail and made a nasty mess of his left thumb. We met at the surgery, for the first time, just a little while later.

Our paths hadn't crossed before since his parish is way over on the other side of Heddington. The Heddington surgery was not open on the Saturday of the thumb-splitting, so on the advice of several of his parishioners who were also patients of mine, Father Padraig arranged to be driven over to see me.

He must have been in a great deal of pain as I drilled a hole in the nail to relieve the pressure, but his only outward sign of discomfort was to mutter under his breath in Latin. I politely apologized for what I was doing but carried on regardless, long ago having recognized that I often earn my living in ways that are unpleasant to others.

Only earlier that same morning, a woman had been brought into the surgery having fallen off her horse and injured her ankle. She was wearing knee-length riding boots that I needed to remove in order to X-ray the underlying damage. Because the injured ankle was already so swollen by the time she arrived, the boot had to be cut away rather than simply pulled off. As I got to work with the shears, the woman burst into tears.

"Am I hurting you?" I asked.

"No," she sobbed, "but those boots were brand-new on this morning, and they cost me a fortune."

"You're a lucky boy," I told Father Padraig as I looked at the X-rays I had taken. "You might be battered and bruised, but there's nothing actually broken."

"Thank the Lord for small mercies," he replied and crossed himself.

"When I went through school, Latin was compulsory," I said later as I was putting the final touches to my bandaging. "As a consequence, I had it pummeled into me over several years by the succession of sadists that my school chose to employ for this task. A lot of it has now faded, of course, but in all of *de Bello Gallico* as well as the various scribblings of Virgil and Cicero, I don't remember coming across any of the words that you've just been muttering."

"Well, you wouldn't have," he said with a twinkle in his eye. "They teach only the common words to Protestants, as I can hear that you are. The really interesting words are reserved for Irish followers of the faith so that they can express their true feelings about English torturers masquerading as medical men who make holes in their thumbs."

"Can I remind you, sir"—I smiled back at him—"that it was you and you alone who swung the hammer!"

"And now," he replied, "you are simply clinging to technicalities."

When Father Padraig reappeared at the surgery the following day after morning mass to have his thumb redressed, he had removed the thumb stall I had provided and replaced it with a black one.

"Very natty," I said admiringly.

"Well," he replied, "a man in my position has to keep up his standards. If I'd let myself wear the white thumb stall you provided while preaching the words of the Lord, who knows what deprivations the congregation might be tempted to stoop to."

■ ■ ■

"Would the Englishman like to come around for dinner?" Father Padraig phoned the surgery a few weeks after I returned to from my sick leave and asked. "He has heard me yattering on about my finches so much that I thought he might like to actually come over and see them."

"I'm sure that would be lovely," Heather said on my behalf, and a few days later, after the surgery had closed for the day, I drove over to Heddington. My knock at the door was answered by a lady in a long black dress with a white lace collar. She might have stepped straight out of *American Gothic*, except that she was smiling. Behind her stood two large wolves that were snarling at me and dripping saliva on the tiled floor.

"Follow me," she said brightly.

"But what about..." I said, gesturing at her friends.

"Oh, don't worry yourself about them. You'll be all right as long as you stay close to me," she replied, and I have never walked as close to anyone as I did to her on our way through to the dining room.

"Just don't make eye contact with them," she said over her shoulder. I followed the instructions to the letter but, like Orpheus before me, found it surprisingly difficult not to look back. Especially at beasts that sounded as if they are weighing up exactly how best to rip me to pieces.

As we entered the dining room, Father Padraig rose from his chair and greeted me in his usual hearty manner.

"I see you have already met Magdalena, my housekeeper," he said. "She has been with me for over twenty years, and I don't know what I'd do without her," he said, rubbing his rather large tummy. "And just as well that I found her," he continued, "for I don't think that anybody else would have put up with me."

Then he put a hand on each of the dogs. "I would also like to introduce you to Ignatius and Benedict," he continued. Apparently, they were Iggy and Ben to their friends.

"They scared the living daylights out of me," I said.

"Don't worry, they're just pussycats," he said, but the dogs were still snarling and dripping, and I wasn't the slightest bit convinced.

"I had a patient once," I replied, "a dear sweet old thing who had some cats. I went to do a house call on her one day and found that they'd mauled her to death by them. There were pieces of her scattered all over the place."

Father Padraig looked at me sideways for just a second and then threw back his head and laughed. "Come on, Mr. Storyteller," he said. "Whilst Magdalena is getting ready to serve up our evening meal, you and I will go and have a look at the birds before it gets dark."

It was a really enjoyable interlude. Father Padraig knew a great deal about his breeding program, and by the end of the tour, I had brushed the cobwebs off a great deal of long-neglected genetics.

That evening is still fresh in my mind. The three of us joked and drank and ate and joked, and later on, I even nervously stroked the wolves. I can't remember exactly what we discussed that night, but I do remember a feeling of being cared for. There were supportive inquiries into my recently restored health, and strong advice about, not overdoing it at the surgery again.

Although I didn't see a great deal of Father Padraig because of the distance between Dixon's Bridge and Heddington, that never seemed to matter. We developed one of those friendships that immediately picks up from wherever it has left off, irrespective of how much sand has trickled through the hourglass in the meantime. From time to time, Father Padraig would come over and see me at the surgery, and from time to time, Magdalena would phone with an invitation for dinner. I always enjoyed the visits but never learned to fully relax around Iggy and Ben. Much as I tried to be friendly, they forever looked at me as if they were wondering what I tasted like. One night Father Padraig dined at Woongarra, and I made him my salmon dish. The evening was pleasant enough, but once, he made it quite clear, was going to be quite enough for him.

"Whilst most fare pales into insipid insignificance when compared to Magdalena's offerings," he had said as he left, "your cooking is *non gratum anus rodentum.*"

▪ ▪ ▪

One evening surgery, not long before Christmas, Meaghan passed on a message from Father Padraig, asking if I would like to go over to Heddington when I had finished the surgery, but to meet him at the church instead of the house. It was a dirty night, and I was dog-tired, and if it hadn't been for the slightly unusual nature of the request, I might have excused myself.

I arrived to find the church lit up like a beacon. I walked in and found Father Padraig sitting on the altar steps.

"Good to see you, boyo," he greeted me breezily without getting up. "Come over and have some of this wine," he said, gesturing to the half-empty decanter on the step next to him, "Which I am happy to assure you, is surplus to the needs of the congregation."

"Are you okay?" I asked as I sat down.

"Never been better," he said and poured me a glass.

"Come on," I said, "what's up?"

"Just fancied some company," he replied. "That's all."

"I'll try again," I said when we had drained our glasses. "What's up?"

He paused for a long time before answering. "If there's anything up," he finally said as he gestured at the church around us, "it's all this."

Father Padraig's parish boasts a particularly lovely church dating back to the gold rush days, and I couldn't see what he was talking about.

"All what?" I replied as I looked around.

"I love my parishioners, and I see it as a privilege to serve them," he replied. "There's no problem with any of that. Where the problem is, is that I've come to wonder whether all of this"—and he gestured at the church again—"assists me in my work or gets in the way of it. I mean, look at you," he continued. "All you have to do is put on a white coat and hang a plastic toy round your neck, and the world immediately follows wherever you lead."

"But everyone thinks that you're a cross between Saint Christopher, King Solomon, and—" I started to reply.

"Yes, but—" he interrupted and then paused.

For a moment, I thought he was going to continue, but he didn't. He closed his mouth, took off his serious face and smiled. "Well, enough of all of that," he eventually continued. "Have a little more of our Savior's blood with me—that is, as long as you've taken your confirmation."

"Well, as a matter of fact, I have," I replied smugly.

Confirmation classes hadn't really been my fourteen-year-old cup of tea, but at my mother's insistence, I had reluctantly promised to attend the first session. It turned out to be an incomprehensibly boring presentation on the sanctity of human relationships. I was on the point of deciding that, whatever my mother might say,

I would not be coming to any further classes when Ruth, the girl sitting directly behind me, leaned forward and gently tapped me on the shoulder. She whispered in my ear that if we went around to the back of the church after the meeting, she would let me touch her breasts, and I astounded my parents with an unfailing willingness to attend the rest of the course.

"The Lord works in mysterious ways," Father Padraig roared laughing and refilled our glasses.

As I was making my farewell, a little later on that evening, Father Padraig asked if I would like to come over and join him for the Christmas day service.

"The congregation can sometimes get a little sleepy, what with all that Christmas pudding and turkey inside them," he said, "and having an English protestant in their midst would make them sit up and pay attention."

"Well, okay then, I will," I replied, and on the spur of the moment, added, "and what's more, I'll bring my mother along with me."

Father Padraig leaned forward and narrowed his eyes. "Wonderful." He smiled. "If I could convert the chairperson of the Anglican Women's Guild to Catholicism, wouldn't that just guarantee me a gold-plated seat slap bang next to Peter."

Later that evening, at home, I phoned my mother.

"I'd like to take you to church on Christmas day," I said.

"Really?" she said in surprise. "Well, that would be lovely, dear. I shall look forward to that."

Christmas day was a shocker. Despite it being summer, the day was cold and gloomy, and gusts of wind drove sheets of rain before them. When my mother arrived up from town, she was running late because of the weather. We briefly exchanged season's greetings and then headed straight off.

As we drove through Dixon's Bridge, we passed the road to the Anglican church. "You've missed the turning, Paul," my mother said.

"No, I haven't," I replied with a smile, and headed up the Heddington road.

"Where are we going?" she asked.

"Secret," I replied.

"Well, I just hope it's not one of those odd churches where they clap," she said and then sat in silent apprehension until twenty minutes later, having crossed the divide, we pulled up in front of the Immaculate Conception of the Holy Mary Mother of God.

"I can't go in there," my mother said in horror.

"Why on earth not," I said. "It's the same God, isn't it?"

"Well, I'm not so sure about that," she spluttered as I helped her out of the car and held up an umbrella to give her protection against the wind and the rain. We hurried up the path, and were just in time, for as we reached the church door, the storm really let fly. At the very moment of our entry, there was a vivid bolt of lightning behind us and a terrific clap of thunder.

We settled ourselves down among the congregation, and I nodded around to various people who I recognized. Just a few minutes later, Father Padraig appeared, and proceedings got under way. The service was delightful, and my mother was pleasantly surprised to find that Catholics sing the same hymns as Protestants and even read from the same Bible.

Father Padraig's sermon was great fun. He has the gift of gab, and his joke about the three men who arrived at the pearly gates on Christmas morning filled the church with laughter. As he was winding up, he said, "Many of you will realize that we have Dr. Carter and his mother with us today. It is delightful to see them, but I am not sure whether the son et lumiere that our Maker organized for their entrance was to signify their conversion to the true faith or simply to warn the rest of us that they had arrived."

At nibbles and wine with Father Padraig in the rectory after the service, my mother was quite overwhelmed by his charm.

"What a lovely, lovely man," she kept saying on the way back. "His service was so genuine. No wonder he has such a large congregation."

"But I thought he worshipped a false god," I teased.

My mother thoroughly enjoyed her naughtiness that Christmas but, to this very day, has kept her visit to the dark side a secret. She laughs and jokes about it with me from time to time, and occasionally even asks me to convey her best wishes to Father Padraig, but she has never repeated the exercise.

■ ■ ■

One late afternoon toward the end of the summer, having a pre-dinner stroll around the aviary once more, our talk got around to bushwalking. Father Padraig came up with the idea that we should go for a stroll along the Howqua river. It seemed that he knew the country up there well and would like to show me some of his favorite places. There and then, we decided that before Easter overwhelmed his calendar, we would load up the pickup with hiking gear and head off for the high country.

■ ■ ■

Although it was already bitterly cold in the mountains, we had a terrific time. We walked along the banks of icy rivers and stayed in some of the various huts that are dotted throughout the valleys. We chatted with other walkers along the way, and over the course of the weekend, finished off the bottle of Irish whisky that Father Padraig had taken along "strictly for medicinal purposes."

"Did you always want to go into the church?" I asked one evening over the campfire.

"To be sure, and it wasn't like that at all." He laughed. "There was never any question. There were six of us boys, and right from the start, me mam had it all organized. David did obstetrics, to bring us all into the world. Michael went into architecture, so that everyone would have a roof over their head. Peter became an engineer, to keep everything running. James did law, to check there was no foul play. And I was sent into the church, to make sure that everyone got ready for the hereafter."

"Hang on," I said, "that's only five."

"And there was also Finn," he continued, "who became the black sheep of the family, just to keep the rest of us on our toes."

"And was he good at it?" I asked.

"The very best," Father Padraig replied with a smile. "If he wasn't getting out of a scrape, he was getting into one. He would be poor one minute and filthy rich the next. He would lose everything on the ponies, borrow from the family to make ends meet, and then cause great dramas by never paying it back. And he would bring both his girlfriend as well as his wife to family gatherings. And the star-spangled wonder of it all was that he got away with it. To avoid any public disgrace, the family simply covered up for him. I thought he was Cú Chulainn and Fionn mac Cumhaill all rolled into one."

"Any girls?" I asked.

"Of course," he replied. "There were six of them too. From the top they did nursing, teaching, and orders, and then the younger ones also did nursing, teaching, and orders. A great one for symmetry, me mam was," he added.

"So what more were you going to say to me that night on the altar steps?" I asked a little later on in the evening.

"Don't you worry your little shiny pate over that," he said after a moment's thought. "We've come up here to get away from all of that and to commune directly with nature. With nothing in between. With nothing getting in the way. So let us do just that."

I confess I was a little disappointed, for I would have liked to hear more of his thoughts on what gets in the way of what. To change the subject, however, I asked his views on how best to solve the tug-of-war between fulfilling the needs of others while, at the same time, safeguarding one's own.

"Despite all that has happened, I still struggle with balancing looking after myself, and looking after my patients," I said and went on to tell him how busy the practice was and how impossible it seemed to do anything about it. I also told him how much I was missing Helen. It felt good opening up to him, and it was a good while before I finished.

He gazed silently into the embers for a few moments. "We all have to find our own way, Paul," he eventually replied, "but I will tell you a story that might help. Recently, a parishioner came up to me after I'd given a sermon on the importance of living for today, whilst still keeping half an eye on getting ready for eternity, you understand. The man thanked me for my words and then told me that he had recently come to realize that life is like a soap dispenser. 'You can never see how much there is left,' he said, 'and then one day you press the button and nothing comes out.'"

I looked over at Father Padraig to see if he was being serious. He wasn't, so we both laughed.

▪ ▪ ▪

I didn't see Father Padraig for some time after our walk. With winter coming on, I was even more overrun in the surgery, and it was a busy time for him too. Then one evening, while having a reunion dinner with the Gentlemen's eleven at the Broken Wheel, I was interrupted by our host, who informed that there was a phone call for me at reception. It was Heather on the line. She asked if I could go urgently to the rectory at Heddington.

"Magdalena called me," she explained. "Apparently, the GP over there is away."

"Yes, but how did you know where—" I started to say.

"She thinks Father Padraig's having a heart attack," she cut in.

"Of course, of course," I replied. "Could you please organize an ambulance to meet me there?" I asked. I then made my excuses to the rest of the team and shot out of the door.

The Broken Wheel is not far from Heddington, and I was the first to arrive at the rectory. Magdalena was at the door and showed me up to the bedroom. Father Padraig, looking pale and frightened, waved a feeble greeting.

"I'm not going to die, am I?" he asked.

"You are," I said, "just like the rest of us, but the trick is to put it off for as long as possible."

As I listened to the story, I agreed with Magdalena's diagnosis. I gave Father Padraig a spray under his tongue and a shot of morphine in his arm, and just a few minutes later, he was looking and feeling much better.

"The accurate answer to your earlier question," I said as I checked him over again, "is probably not just now, and especially if we can get you off to the hospital in the near future."

"Thank goodness," he replied with a wan smile.

"I've just phoned, and the ambulance will be here in five minutes," Magdalena came in and said.

"Excellent," I said as I turned to her. "In that case, we just have enough time."

"Time for what?" she asked.

"Well, whilst what other people think of you might be none of your business," I continued, "that doesn't mean that you have to keep everyone informed about everything you do."

"What on earth are you talking about?" she asked.

"Although most ambulance officers are confidential and discreet people," I said, "it is just possible that we might be unlucky enough to strike a gossiper. But if we start right now and are quick about it, we'll be able to get all of your stuff out of this room before anyone arrives."

"Oh!" she exclaimed, turning red.

"I'll give you a hand," I said, and while she grabbed all her clothes from the chair in the corner, I cleared everything from the top of the dressing table.

In no time at all, the job was done. As we had a final look round the room to make sure that nothing had been missed, we heard a siren coming down the street. A moment later, two bright and cheerful ambulance officers burst into the room like a whirlwind, connected Father Padraig to an oxygen bottle, loaded him onto a stretcher, and whisked him off to hospital.

After they had left, Magdalena and I went downstairs and had a cup of tea. "Thank you," she simply said as I was leaving.

"Don't mention it," I replied and drove back to the Broken Wheel, but the rest of the boys had already left.

■ ■ ■

After a week or so in hospital, Father Padraig and Magdalena convalesced somewhere down on the coast at a place that belongs to the church. I didn't see him until after his return, and when he came into the surgery for a checkup, I hardly recognized him. He looked fantastic. He must have lost at least forty pounds in weight, and the sea air had put some much-needed color back into his complexion.

"Are you doing anything this evening?" he asked me.

"Nothing special," I replied.

"Well, come on over after your surgery then and have a glass of altar wine with me," he said. "I'll get Magdalena to rustle us up some food."

I got to Heddington at around seven o'clock, and Father Padraig chattered away for a while about his experiences during his hospital stay. When he eventually finished, it was my turn.

"On the night of your heart attack," I said, "and I hope you don't mind me saying this, but especially for a man in your position, you seemed mightily worried about the possibility of meeting your Maker."

Father Padraig looked at the ground for a while and didn't say a word. He was quiet for so long that I thought I might have overstepped the mark and offended him. Then he looked up at me. "I'm afraid that I haven't believed in any of all that for a very long time," he said. "I love my congregation, and I love what I do for them, but these days I see things very differently from how I used to."

"I rather suspect," he continued as he gestured around us, "that this is all that we get, but that has never stopped me wanting to help those who believe that it's not."

There was another long pause, and then he continued. "And about your visit. Magdalena has looked after me for many years, and we have long known that we had feelings for one another. A year ago, Magdalena found out that she had cancer, and since, even now, no one is able to tell us how long she has left, we changed our relationship."

■ ■ ■

I was in a very reflective mood when I got home that night. Nel was waiting for me by the back door, and when I asked if she would sit up and chat for a while, she happily agreed.

"Do you think that a life of selfless caring for others is especially wonderful in the face of doubts about one's own personal beliefs?" I asked her. "And do you think it even more powerful when that care is given as a deliberate choice rather than simply from any sense of duty?"

Nel sat and looked silently up at me for quite some time.

"Je n'ai pas la moindre idée de ce que tu dit,"[21] she eventually said and then curled up in her bed and went back to sleep.

21. I haven't the faintest idea what you're talking about.

RECIPES FOR DISASTER

Saumon Fromage

1 tin of salmon
½ tub cream cheese
3 shakes Tabasco
½ egg cup lemon juice

1. Mix salmon and cream cheese.
2. Add Tabasco and lemon.
3. Mix again.

17

MUNG

Beyond the farmyard, down by the shearing shed, stands a tiny weatherboard cottage. Mrs. Smith had lived in it for many decades and only left with my arrival. She had "let the garden go," as she put it. She had also added her own stamp to the tangled jungle, which sprang up around her abode, by disposing of her household rubbish through the simple expedient of throwing it out of whichever window happened to be the closest at the time. The place looked like a huge rubbish tip with an old growth forest poking out of the top.

There was an avalanche of jobs to be done on the farm in the early days, and since I was also very busy in the practice, things only got done on the basis of urgent need. As the cottage was hidden from everyday view, it was not a high priority, and for many years things stayed much as they were when I first arrived. But nothing stays the same forever. There came a time when rats started promenading on top of the rubbish piles in broad daylight, and I decided that the time had obviously arrived for something to be done. The rubbish pile had to go.

It was suggested to me that I seek the services of Mung for this sort of work, so I phoned him up and organized for him to come around and clear away the mess. Mung, who is built much along the lines of a bowling ball and has even less hair than I do, is a talented artist with a Bobcat. In just a few days of taking many truckloads of rubbish to the tip, and a massive bonfire that, for a short but exciting period of time, almost got away from us, I became the proud owner of a tiny dilapidated cottage standing in the middle of a clearing of broken ground littered with a thin scattering of Mrs. Smith's leftovers.

"There you go," Mung said as he looked at his handiwork with pride, "as smooth as a baby's bum."

The whole job went really well until the very last day. It was then that Mung climbed onto the top of his machine, chainsaw in hand, to knock off a few final overhanging branches that were getting in his way. In reaching for the last one, he had stepped into thin air.

On the way down, Mung's forearm came in contact with, first, the chainsaw and then the ground.

I was working round the back of the cottage at the time and didn't see the accident. I heard the cry for help, however, and raced round at high speed. I wrapped Mung's arm in a towel, put him in my pickup, and drove him to the clinic.

"It's not been a good day," he said as we traveled along. "I've lost my teeth as well."

"What, just now when you fell?" I asked.

"No," he replied. "I recently got myself a new pup, and the little bugger's hidden 'em somewhere in my garden. I only got 'em a week or so ago, and they fit real well. Got 'em especially for my wedding." He grinned coyly.

"I didn't know you'd just got married," I said as we reached the clinic. "Congratulations," I added. As I cleaned his arm, ready for doing some embroidery, I unearthed an armful of tattoos.

"What is this one on your forearm meant to be?" I asked, looking at a picture that straddled the wound.

"A ship's rigging," he replied.

"And so it is," I said as I leaned forward, "but it looks as if it's been through a hell of a battle."

"It was fine when it was done. You're the one who buggered it up," he said to my surprise.

I had no idea what he was talking about at first, but as I looked down at the battered rigging, memories returned, and I realized that this would not be the first time that I had sewn up Mung's arm.

Very early on a Sunday morning many years before, I had been called out of my nice, warm bed to see a young man who had fallen through a plate glass window at his parents' thirtieth wedding anniversary.

Before heading off to the surgery, I phoned Leslie and asked if she could possibly meet me at the clinic to give me a hand. In the event, she arrived ahead of me, and I waved her a "thank you" to her as I pushed my way through the large and noisy crowd who had come along to top off their evening's entertainment.

When I finally managed to fight my way to the center of the action, I found a lad lying on the examination couch with his right arm swathed in a huge bundle of bloodstained towels. There was also a large red stain over much of his clothes, and yet more sprayed out when Leslie and I started to unravel the towels to have a better look.

We quickly put them back in place again, and I popped in a drip on the other side.

"What's your name, son?" I asked.

"Mung," he slurred.

"And where are your parents?"

"Buggered if I know," he slurred again.

I cut the sleeve off his shirt and put on a tourniquet. I then carefully removed the towels again, revealing a large tattoo of a four-master running before the wind, with a large cut running through the middle of it. I also found that, in addition to making a mess of the four-master, Mung had snagged a fair-sized blood vessel into the bargain.

It was a tricky repair, for I was constantly bumped in the back by well-wishers hoping for a better view, and Mung repeatedly and tunelessly sang "Good old Collingwood forever" in my ear.

When I eventually finished and stood up to stretch my back, the treatment room door opened, and Dale, Mung's father, came in. He strode over to his son, looked down at him for a moment, and then turned to me. I smiled at him, imagining that I was about to get a pat on the back.

"He won't be happy with that, you know," Dale said.

"What?" I said in disbelief.

"No, he won't be happy with that at all," he said. "Mung's always been very fussy about his appearance. You can tell that by the jeans he wears. And that," Dale said as he picked up the sleeve I'd cut off, "was a new shirt on this evening."

Before I could reply, the door opened for a second time, and Edith, Mung's other parent, also squeezed in. She pushed her way through the crowd and took me by the hands.

"I am delighted to report that the arm is going to be fine," I started to say, but she cut across me before I'd said so much as a word.

"Doc," she said, "you won't forget to write him out a work certificate for Monday, will you? His boss can get very narky about things like that," and without another word, she turned and left.

Later, when the crowd were finally dispersing, Kaz, Mung's baby sister, tapped me on the shoulder. "There's another thing Mung won't be happy about," she said and pointed at her brother's arm. "You didn't get his rigging lined up."

"Oh," I said, and now that she mentioned it, I could see that I hadn't.

■ ■ ■

Chainsaws make a lot of damage when they come in contact with human anatomy. Mung's arm was no exception, and it took quite a while to work out which bits went where. As I toiled away, Mung asked if I'd ever seen any chainsaw wounds before.

"Chainsaws," I said, "have provided me with a regular income for many years," and when he pressed me for details, I told him about the fellow who had been cutting up a branch while holding it in place with his foot.

"But everyone does that," Mung said.

"I know," I replied, "but not in the pouring rain when you're only wearing thongs, so that when you slip, the saw goes straight into your shin, and most of the way through."

Mung screwed up his face at the story, so I decided not to tell him about the locum priest who'd come up to Dixon's Bridge only the year before to stand in for one of the local pastors while he took some time off.

There was an old tree overhanging the vestry of the church that the stand-in was looking after. Being a tall man, he banged his head on it every time he went in and out and, after a day or two, decided to do something about it. He found a chainsaw in the shed, filled it with fuel, and managed to get it going. He then went back to the vestry, opened the throttle, and reached up as high as he could to cut off the offending limb.

I am not sure if he was experienced with chainsaws or not. Either way, he neglected to put on the helmet that was sitting on the bench beside the saw, which was a pity, for when the chain hit the underlying brickwork and ricocheted back, it took him full in the face.

I eventually finished Mung's repair and then stood back and looked at the results of my handiwork. "There you go," I said, "as smooth as a baby's bum."

▪ ▪ ▪

From time to time, Mung comes up to Woongarra for a day's work. There are always drains to be cleaned, driveways to be patched up, or stumps to be pulled. Mung does it all well, and I enjoy working with him.

"You should come over and have a look at my place one day," he said when we were having a spot of lunch together.

"I will at that," I replied, and the following weekend, when all the chores had got themselves finished earlier than expected, I did.

Mung lives high up on Mount Miranda, and not having visited the place before, I was very impressed. Although the house itself is quite modest, on one side it is joined directly to an enormous bird cage and, on the other side, to an equally impressive structure, the purpose of which is not immediately obvious to the first-time visitor. But what really catches the eye is the open- sided hayshed that stands over the whole complex, dominating the skyline.

"Come on in," Mung greeted me with a wide smile. "Let me show you around."

"Goodness," I said as he opened a door from the family room, and we walked straight into a huge aviary. It was a world of noise and activity, and we were immediately surrounded by a kaleidoscope of color and flapping wings. There were birds everywhere, and they settled on Mung in surprisingly large numbers as soon as he appeared, nibbling at his ears and jumper.

"Come to Daddy," he said and made kissing noises at them. "Pretty good, eh," he said from out of a halo of parrots.

"Fantastic," I replied.

"And what's on the other side of the house?" I asked after Mung eventually shook off his admirers.

"I'll show you," he replied, and we crossed back through the house. This time we exited through the laundry door, and as we did so, I found myself looking eyeball to eyeball with a monitor lizard, much the same size as myself, that was lying in the fork of a tree.

"Don't worry," Mung laughed as I jumped back, "she'd lick you to death rather than have a go at you," but I decided not to put it to the test.

Like the aviary, the lizardarium was as big as the house, and also like the aviary, there were plenty of residents. Apart from the one that had said hello to me when I came in, they were everywhere, and they were huge. They were lying on top of logs, lying under logs, lying around the pool, and some were even glued to the walls.

"Doesn't it get a bit cold up here for these fellows?" I asked as I looked around admiringly.

"That's why I let them inside," he said. "But they're a bloody nuisance. I try to keep them in the family room, but they're always escaping, and we find them all over the place. Kaz won't come here since she found one in her bed."

"The whole setup's fantastic," I said as we went back into the house. "But just one thing," I added, "what's with the hay shed?"

"Oh, you noticed," he replied. "Well, the house was leaking like a sieve, but when I got a quote for doing the repairs, it was ridiculous. The birds and lizards were often getting knocked about by the weather anyway, so I decided to just put a shed over the whole thing. It was much cheaper, and I got my picture in the paper an' all when I did it. I always thought the idea might catch on."

"It nearly did," I said.

"Did it?" he said. "Well, there you go."

"Who's that working out in the garden?" I asked, looking out of the kitchen window.

"That's my wife and her sister," he said. We were about to go outside to say hello when the ladies in question stood up, waved, and came indoors, carrying baskets full of vegetables.

"My wife, Sumalee, and her sister, Tika," Mung introduced proudly when they had put their things down, and I was presented to the two tiniest ladies I have ever met.

"Delighted to meet you," I said, but they just smiled back without saying anything.

"They're not so hot on the English," Mung explained, so I simply bowed.

"So how did you two meet?" I asked a little later as we sipped some tea.

"I went over there on a holiday," Mung replied. "Met her through a friend back here who's married to her cousin. It was love at first sight," he added. "We even got married twice, once over there and then again once back here."

"I hope you don't mind me asking," he continued after a pause, "but now that you're on the mend again, do you think you'll ever have another go at getting married?"

"Well, yes, I hope so," I said and told him that I even had someone in mind.

"So what's holding you back?" he asked.

"She's in France," I said a little sadly.

"Really? Why wouldn't you just pick someone nearer to home?" he asked.

"Because she's the one for me," I replied a little sadly.

"And how do you know that?" he asked.

"Because I've been in love with her most of my life," I replied.

In answer to Mung's puzzled expression, I explained that I'd recently had my sitting room redecorated. The evening before the painters were due to start, I had moved everything out of the room, including all the books from the bookshelves, to give them room to work. It was a long and tiring chore, and partway through the evening, feeling hungry and thirsty, I'd stopped for a drop of the hard stuff and made myself some egg and chicks. While I was having my break, I had idly looked at some of the books I had stacked on the table. They were a collection of ones I had enjoyed as a teenager, and when I came across *Ayesha*, I casually flicked it open.

To my total surprise, on a fly leaf just inside the front cover, there was a picture of Helen. I was stunned. She was floating above the earth and dressed only in the flimsiest of costumes. Suddenly, I was fourteen again, and just like then, I couldn't take my eyes off her.

"I have an idea," Mung continued as if I hadn't spoken. "France is a helluva long way from here. How about Tika? All you've got to do is say the word, and I'll arrange everything for you. I mean, they're really grouse, these sheilas, and they look after you real nice. They work hard, and they never whinge like Australian women. I should know, I was married to one once, and I swore I'd never make that mistake again. Would you like us to leave the two of you alone for a bit to get to know one another?" Mung asked.

"Well," I said with a faint smile, "that's a really kind offer, but I don't think so."

Tika looked like a perfectly nice person, but quite apart from Helen's ability to float above the earth in flimsy costumes, I had always imagined myself spending the future with someone I could have a conversation with.

▪ ▪ ▪

I didn't see Mung for quite a while after that, and thought that he and Sumalee might have gone up north in search of the sun. Then one afternoon, he was brought into the surgery, having injured himself yet again. Apparently, he had rolled his Bobcat on a slope while clearing fallen timber on a neighbor's property. From all accounts, he'd been lucky to get out of it alive.

"Made a real mess of the Bobcat," he said.

"Your arm's not looking that flash either," I replied as Leslie and I scraped away the dirt and exposed another large gash.

"By the way, if you're wanting to get married," Mung said as I put in the local, "that offer of mine's still on the table."

"Thanks, but no thanks," I replied as Leslie looked up at me quizzically from the other side of Mung's arm. "I'll explain it later," I said to her.

When the arm was ready for repair, I realized that the new wound was right over where I'd repaired the arm twice before.

"You've made a mess of my old handiwork," I observed.

"Have I?" he said, looking down at his arm. "How lucky can you get?"

"And how's that?" I asked.

"It'll give you a chance to straighten up the dog's breakfast you made of it twice before," he said. "See if you can get the rigging sorted out this time," he continued, "there's a good lad," and I promised to do my best.

RECIPES FOR DISASTER

Egg and Chicks

1 egg
6 chicken wings
¼ jar vegemite

1. Fry the egg on one side of the pan.
2. Fry the chicken wings on the other.
3. Serve on toast with vegemite.

18

FRATELLI

With Helen still overseas, many people felt that I needed an interest outside of the surgery to help in my continuing recovery. I was invited to join the local bowls club, and although I won a frozen chicken at the novice's night, I decided that the game wasn't really my cup of tea. The same went for Rotary and the local historical society. Both lovely groups of people but, again, not what I was looking for.

I finally decided that I'd like to get back into music, and I pulled out and dusted off the clarinet that had been sitting in the bottom of a cupboard for many a long year. To my great disappointment, I found that whatever talent I might have possessed in my youth had long since evaporated. All I got out of my licorice stick were a few squeaks and lips so sore that it took several days before I could speak properly again.

"Why not learn the piano?" Meaghan asked at morning tea, and the seed was sown.

"Why not indeed," I replied. After all, I'd seen Bill Murray do it in *Groundhog Day*, and it looked easy enough.

"It shouldn't take us long." I smiled at Emily, a local teacher. "I only want to learn the Rach three and the Hummel A minor, and I already know that the black notes play louder than the white ones."

"Very funny." She smiled back.

"You're terrible, Muriel." She smiled at me again at the end of the first lesson. "Have you got anything to practice on?" she asked, and when I answered in the negative, she told me I had better find something.

▪ ▪ ▪

A few evenings later, I happened to do a house call on Constanza, the matriarch of a large local Italian family, all of whose members I knew well. She had a dreadful chest infection and wasn't well enough to come to the surgery. At the start of the visit, it was just Constanza and me, but as had happened before when her husband, Mario, broke his leg and I visited him at home, gradually the entire family drifted in by ones and twos. By the time I finished the clinical side of things and was drinking a cup of eye-watering coffee that made my tongue stick to the roof of my mouth, the room was packed.

When I happened to mention that I was looking for a piano, there was an immediate chorus of offers of help. It was agreed by one and by all that my needs could most easily be met by Enzo, a cousin who restored and sold pianos out of the old fire station at Cowley. Mario assured me that the family would see to it that I was well looked after.

As a result, the next time I managed to get away from the surgery early, I went over to Cowley to have a look and see what was on offer.

On the way over, I imagined that I would spend a pleasant half hour chatting with Enzo, choose an unpretentious upright, and then go home and wait for it to be delivered. What actually happened was that Enzo and I talked until it was time to close the shop, and then went back to his place for a meal. After we had eaten, my host then spent the rest of the evening giving me a blow-by-blow account of his love life over the previous ten years. It certainly contained some surprises for I recognized the names of several of my regulars.

Somewhere around one o'clock and close to the bottom of the second, or maybe the third, bottle of red, I bought a baby grand off him.

"It's in perfect working order." Enzo smiled his dazzling perfect smile, and just over a week later, it was sitting in the middle of my living room.

To my surprise, I enjoyed practicing each night when I got home from work. I also knew that I was making progress when Nel, instead of scratching at the back door to be let out as soon as I started, began sitting next to me and singing along.

I was a bit disappointed, however, for although the piano had sounded just fine with Enzo at the keyboard, it didn't sound nearly as good with me there. I decided that although I'd only had the instrument for a few weeks, perhaps it needed a tune.

I couldn't get hold of Enzo, who was out of the district, apparently avoiding someone's husband, so I mentioned my need to Mario.

"No aproblem," he said and gave me the telephone number of Umberto, another cousin who made his living going around to people's houses, doing exactly what I needed.

"Where does he live?" I asked when I didn't recognize the area code, so Mario told me.

"Deniliquin!" I exclaimed. "That's the other side of the moon."

"It's no aproblem," Mario continued without interruption. "He acomes down all atime."

Following Mario's advice, I phoned Umberto and arranged a date for him to visit.

"Vot time vould you like me to arrive?" he asked and broke off into a coughing fit.

"Let's get off to a bright start. How about nine o'clock?" I suggested, and I think he said yes, although with all the spluttering it was hard to tell.

"Are you okay?" I asked when he eventually got his breath back, and he assured me that he was.

Having looked forward with anticipation to Umberto's visit, I was more than a little disappointed when he didn't arrive. After an hour or so of sitting around waiting for him, I decided it would be pointless to hang on for any longer and went off and got on with some of the jobs around the place that I had been putting off for some time.

By late evening, I was just thinking about having an early night when there was a knock at the front door. I answered it to find a tiny wizened old man standing on the doorstep. There was a battered old two-tone station wagon in the driveway behind him.

"Gut efening," he wheezed as he shook my hand. "I am Umberto. I beleef you zed nine o'clock. Inconvenient and unusual"—he smiled at me—"but ve vish to please and haf made it just on time."

"Oh! I'd imagined that we'd meant…" I started to say and was about to state the obvious when two other people stepped out of the car.

"Zis," Umberto said as he introduced me to a large islander lady in her late twenties, "is my wife, Clementine, and zis," he continued as I shook hands with an equally elderly man who should clearly have pursued a career as a basketball player, "is my apprentice, Raymond."

"Do you haf any food?" Umberto asked when the three of them had come inside. "Ve haf been on ze road all day, and ve are very hungry." So I rustled up some beans on toast while they went back out and brought in all their gear from the car.

"Wow," I said when I saw the pile they had made in the hall. "Will you be able to get everything finished tonight?" I asked.

"Oh no." Umberto laughed. "It is too late to start now. Ve von't do anything tonight. Ve vill start first zing in ze morning."

"So where are you staying?" I asked.

"Vell, here, of course," he said, "Vere else?" and they all smiled at me. "Und since Clementine and I no longer share a bed, you know, ve vill need three rooms," so I spent the next twenty minutes stretching the meager contents of my linen cupboard as far as they would go. When I got back to the kitchen, the three of them were helping themselves to a bottle of wine they'd found in the fridge.

"Vould you like a little nightcap?" Umberto smiled at me and offered some of my own dry white.

For a split second, I thought of kicking up a fuss, but then I simply said, “Yes, okay, I don’t mind if I do.”

“On ze vay down, I vas just talking about ze war,” Umberto said as he sipped between coughs. “Ven the Germans took over Italy, I had to tune many of their pianos. Once even for a concert for Goebbels. I had to be very careful, of course,” he added.

“I could imagine he would have been pretty fussy,” I replied.

“He vos,” Umberto answered, “but my need for care was mostly because I should haf been vearing a star. Zat vas ven I learned to speak with a German accent, of course,” he added.

And as late evening turned into early morning, I learnt that Umberto was the world’s leading expert on Wurlitzers, spoke seven different languages, had been involved in everything from the Berlin Philharmonic to Barbershop Quartets and had married Clementine only the year before. I don’t think anyone else got a word in edgewise, and we all decided it was time to retire when there was no more wine left in the fridge.

As we were heading off to our respective bedrooms, Umberto caught sight of the piano. “I vill just have one quick look for you,” he said and sat down at the piano and started to play the *Appasionata.* It sounded pretty good to me, but almost as soon as he began playing, Umberto started frowning. In full flight, he suddenly stopped and lifted the lid.

“Oy vey,” he wheezed as he looked inside. “Zis is not good,” and he beckoned to Raymond, who looked over Umberto’s shoulder and said, “Oh dear, oh dear, *oh dear.*”

“What’s the problem?” I came up behind them and asked apprehensively.

Umberto looked back at me and shook his head. “Zis is very bad.” He shook his head. “Ze strings are all rusted.”

“That’s bad, huh?” I inquired.

“Very bad,” he muttered.

“Very bad indeed,” Raymond agreed.

“Well, I guess we’ll have to get some new strings then,” I said helpfully.

"But for zis piano, zey no longer exist," Umberto answered. "Ve vill haf to make zem by hand, each und everyvon."

"Oh," I said.

"And also the action," he added sadly.

"What?" I exclaimed, and for an answer, he dropped some small pellets into the palm of my hand.

"You haf rodents," he said and then, as he handed me some chewed-up felt, he added, "und zilverfish."

"Oh," I said again. "This is all beginning to sound a bit expensive."

For reply, Umberto looked up at the ceiling and tapped the fingers of one hand on the palm of the other. After a while, he looked back at me and quoted a figure twice as large as I had paid for the piano in the first place. He then bade me good night, leaving me gasping for breath and looking down thoughtfully at a handful of mouse poo and fragments of compressed wool.

Sometime during the night, I was tapped on the shoulder by Clementine. Initially I misunderstood her intentions, but then I realized that she was indicating that she wanted help. I followed her through to Umberto's room where I listened to the old man's wheezy chest, gave him something to ease his breathing, and then went to the kitchen and made him some honey and lemon.

▪ ▪ ▪

None of my visitors was up when I left for work the following morning. They had clearly been active during the day, however, for when I got home that night, I found the entire workings of the piano laid out in neat rows across the living room floor.

"How'd you go?" I asked breezily when I found the three of them lined up on the couch watching television. The news wasn't good, however. Apparently, they had uncovered yet more problems, which would have to be discussed over dinner, and was it possible to have something different tonight as the beans had upset Clementine's tummy.

"Everyone happy with fish?" I asked, and three heads nodded as one.

Because of my concerns over the mounting costs associated with the piano repair, I was personally too distracted to enjoy the meal, but not so Clementine. As she finished her third helping, she looked up at me and said the only word I ever heard her utter.

"Good," she said, and I got quite excited for, as far as I can remember, it remains the only time that my cooking has ever received unsolicited and unqualified praise.

During the meal, Umberto and Raymond largely ignored me and spoke between themselves about the merits of different types of organ stops. As soon as they'd had their fill, however, they got down to business.

"Ze keys," Umberto declared as he helped himself to some of the wine that I'd brought home, "vill have to be remade, and also ze pedals."

"What?" I asked incredulously.

"Humidity," he replied accusingly and, when I looked at him blankly, continued, "you haf let ze humidity in ze concert room vary, my friend."

"I haven't done anything," I said defensively.

"Exactly," he replied as he drained his glass and refilled it again, "zo I'm afraid zat it vill cost you a little more," and when he told me how much, some of my wine went down the wrong way.

"I vill need some money for ze materials," Umberto said when I eventually recovered, and despite my misgivings, by the time we'd retired, I had given him a sizeable check.

Getting ready to go off to work the next morning, I had to take three slow deep breaths, letting myself relax more with each breath that I took. There was not a soul around again, but there was no hot water left, everyone's teeth were in glasses next to the telephone, and the last of the cereal, milk, and bread had disappeared.

That evening, I arrived home anticipating further signs of progress, only to find that my visitors had left and taken all their belongings with them. The floor of the sitting room was completely bare, and when I lifted the lid on the piano, I found that that all the keys had gone as well.

I sat on the piano stool, looking at the empty shell in front of me and thought dark thoughts about the check I had written.

"Monsieur Gullible," Nel teased, and I thought that she'd pretty much got it right.

Over the next week or so, I repeatedly tried to make contact with Umberto, but without success. Either the phone rang out or I was told by Raymond that Umberto couldn't come to the phone right now.

"But what about my piano?" I complained.

"You'll have to speak to Umberto about that," he would say, and I would reply that that's exactly what I was trying to do.

I even toyed with the idea of driving up to Deniliquin, but it is just such a long way.

▪ ▪ ▪

During the time that Umberto was playing hide-and-seek, Mario came into the surgery, worried that his pacemaker wasn't working properly. When I finished checking him over and was able to reassure him that all was well, I also told him about the piano. He initially frowned, but then his face cleared into a smile.

"Don't you aworry." He beamed. "I asort this out afor you."

"Grazie," I said.

"I have amany acousins," he said with a wink, "but you afar more aspecial than athat."

I didn't hear anything back from Mario, but a week later when I got home from work, I knew that someone had been in the house. For over twenty years, I had left the house unlocked during the day, and there had never once been an intruder. I couldn't see anything that had obviously been moved or changed, but I just knew that someone had been there.

"Did you see who it was?" I would have asked Nel, but she had spent the day at the surgery with me, cheering people up in the waiting room. "Perhaps I'm imagining it," I said to her and went through to the kitchen.

After I'd fed and watered the both of us, I poured myself a glass of wine and wandered back into the living room and sat on the piano stool.

I had been sitting there, meditating, for quite some time when I suddenly realized that there was a large table standing in the middle of my dining area.

I went over to have a closer look and stood open-mouthed in amazement. It was magnificent, and it looked exactly like the one in the showroom all that time before. There was a note attached to the top of it.

Up ya kilt
Gaz

"It's a miracle," I whispered to Nel in awe and wondered if it was grounds for beatification.

"That is fantastic," I said to Gaz on the phone a few minutes later. "Thank you so much," and we chatted on for a few minutes about technical matters, as fellow carpenters do.

"So what do I owe you?" I eventually asked.

"We're all square, remember," he replied brightly. "You've already paid."

"Really?" I asked.

"Yep," he said. "All the stain and gear fell off the back of a truck anyway."

"And what was all that crap you said about having it finished in two weeks?" I asked.

"I did. I just didn't tell you which two weeks it would be." He laughed. "Oh, and thanks for seeing Wol again," he added, for only the week before, Poss and Digger had brought him in again for some more eye drops.

"Perhaps his scratching post's in a draft," I suggested.

"Perhaps it is at that," Gaz replied. "I'll try moving it."

After I put the phone down, I stood there marveling at the table for a while and then poured myself another glass with which to toast its maker.

Then I sat back down on the piano stool, sipping away, and humming happily to myself. In an idle gesture, I opened the lid of the piano and nearly dropped my glass.

Some years before, on a trip to Washington, DC, I had visited the National Gallery of Art. I'd had a lovely morning wandering through the various galleries and then, hungry and slightly footsore, I had gone in search of a sandwich. As I rounded a corner by the lifts, I unexpectedly came upon the *Sacrament of the Last Supper* hanging on the wall. I was quite overcome. It's been my favorite Dali since I won a copy of it as an art prize at school, and I hadn't even known that it was in America, let alone in Washington. It was much bigger and more wonderful than I'd expected, and hunger and weary feet forgotten, I had oohed and aahed over it for ages.

Finding that the keys were back in my piano might not have been quite in the same category as running into JC having dinner with his mates in the new world, but it certainly ran it a close second.

Very tentatively, I tapped one of the keys, and to my further astonishment, a clear, clean, and pleasing sound filled the room. I tapped another key and found that the same thing happened again. I lifted the top lid and gazed admiringly at a bright new action with strings that glittered in the late afternoon light.

"Two miracles is grounds for canonization," I informed Nel in a whisper.

As well as a bright new action, there was also an envelope stuffed with money. It was from Enzo, who had apparently just found out that he'd accidentally overcharged me for the piano. He hadn't realized I was family, the note said.

"Well, thanks very much," I said and gratefully tucked it away.

Later that evening, I went around to Mario and Costanza's. It was a good opportunity to check Costanza's chest again, and I wanted to thank Mario for his help. Fortunately, Costanza was recovering well, and after I had checked her out, I stayed on with them for a bite to eat.

"You can ahave some of those asausages you alike, and also some apaint stripper," Mario said with a laugh, brandishing a flagon of his homemade red as the family gradually drifted in once more. "But I'm not aso sure that I alike what you say about it in your abook."

"Anyway, thank you, Mario," I said, "for helping sort out the piano business."

"Oh, that aremind me," he said and picked up a check from behind the clock on the mantlepiece and handed it to me. It was the one I had written out for Umberto.

"But…" I spluttered, a little confused.

"Umberto," Mario said, "he didn't arealize that ayou afamily either."

Whatever misgivings I might previously have had about paint stripper, I enjoyed it that evening, and it wasn't until late that I set off for home.

We were standing by my car when Mario asked me how I liked my new table.

"How on earth do you know about that?" I asked in astonishment.

"Gazza," he replied simply. "He's another acousin."

"Useful having all these cousins." I laughed.

"I might ahave amany acousins," he said as he reached up and put his arm round my shoulders, "but you and me, we're a lot amore than athat. We're abrothers."

I turned the car round and was about to head off when Mario held out his hand and stopped me. He stuck his head in the open car window and before I knew what he was up to, gave me a kiss on the top of my head.

"And when asomeone's abeen ill," he said, "then their abrother's agot to alook after them even abetter."

RECIPES FOR DISASTER

Crispy Fish

1 fillet of fish with skin
1 lettuce

1. Fry fish skin down.
2. Serve on lettuce leaves.

19

EWA

"Good to have you back on deck again and looking well," Hugo said when I was dining with him and Reggy one evening a couple of months after my return. "But everyone can see," he wagged his finger at me, "that you're starting to overdo it again."

"The solution is screamingly obvious," Reggy interjected. "You simply need some help."

"I sure do," I agreed and drained my glass. "And with any luck, someone who's there for the long haul. A Felix replacement, preferably hardworking, good-looking, and intelligent. Just like me, in fact, except maybe with two X chromosomes and more hair," I added.

"You want a woman?" Hugo asked in a puzzled voice.

"Well, yes, I do," I admitted, "and in more ways than one. But what I was meaning just then was as another pair of hands in the practice. For one thing, I am really over doing gynecological examinations on people I then meet socially. Just recently," I continued, "I was at a dinner party in Dixon's Bridge. I looked round the table and thought, 'My god, I've done everyone here.' The same applies to prostates, of course," I added. "But somehow that's different."

A week or so later, while sorting through my usual lunchtime mail, I came across a package that had been forwarded on to me by my friends who live near the trout stream. It contained a resume with the name Ewa Kozlowski printed neatly across the top. Apparently, so the attached note informed me, this was the lady they would have liked me to have met when I was up there, if only I hadn't had to dash away at no notice.

"She trained in Krakow," my friends explained when I phoned to thank them.

"I can imagine she would have done. And she speaks English?" I asked cautiously.

"Improving," they replied. "Definitely improving."

"You don't have a problem with her being Polish, do you?" they asked.

"No, not in the slightest," I replied and went on to tell them how, by odd coincidence, I had recently gone with some friends to the Polish club down in the city. The decor had been circa 1930s, and the food had been circa 1950s. By nine o'clock, every Pole in the place was dancing with their arms wrapped round one another. By ten o'clock, they were all singing, and by eleven o'clock, they were all crying. It had been a wonderful evening.

"Absolutely not," I repeated after I put the phone down because, some years before, having so enjoyed the company of Archie, my first medical student, I'd let the university know that I'd be happy to take on another one. It just so happened that they were urgently in need of a placement, and they sent along Greg.

During one of the brief episodes of detente that occurred toward the end of the Cold War, the Polish authorities decided to allow out of their country those of their citizens who said that they wanted to live in Israel. Greg's parents had jumped at the opportunity and, together with their small son, had found their way to a holding camp in Austria. From there they were moved to Italy, but then, instead of going on to Israel, they used up their remaining money to buy three tickets on the flying kangaroo, which is, of course, what they had planned to do all along.

Greg was ten when he arrived in Australia. Within two years, he was completely fluent in English, the only remaining linguistic problem being his accent, which made him almost impossible to understand. He has got much better over the years, but even to this day, I have to concentrate hard when I'm listening to him on the phone.

By fourteen, he had duxed his school; by seventeen, he had got himself into medical school; and by twenty-one, he was rolling up my driveway in a battered old Ford ready for a six-week dose of country medicine.

Right from the start Greg was a hit. Not only was his clinical knowledge phenomenal, but he was also eager to soak up the more streetwise education that a country practice has to offer. The girls on the front desk fell in love with him from day one, and all the patients followed suit shortly thereafter.

"Helluva nice guy," they would say. "Just a pity we can't understand a bloody word he says."

"Mind you," they would add, "that makes him fit in nicely."

"What do you mean?" I would ask.

"Well, we need a dictionary to understand half of what you go on about as well."

Greg is a professor of radiology these days, and I feel a warm glow of proprietary pride in this achievement. At the time of his visit, I was still taking most of my own X-rays. I used a large and antiquated machine that looked like some crazy leftover from a bygone era, which, of course, is exactly what it was. It took wonderful pictures, however, and it was on this museum piece that Greg cut his teeth.

I am not sure in how many different ways it is possible to take an X-ray incorrectly, but I do know that Greg pushed the boundary into previously uncharted territory. I also believe that his faultless performance these days is entirely due to the fact that he got every possible mistake out of his system in Dixon's Bridge. When he didn't get the mAs setting wrong, he mucked up the kV, and when he got both those right, he failed to load the cassette or used developer instead of fixer.

But a quitter Greg is not, and on the very last day of his stay, he hit the bull's-eye. In helping me to sort out someone who had limped in on crutches, he produced a perfect picture of a spiral fracture of a fibula. There was an aura of triumph about him as he showed me the film, and even then, I suspected that a career had been launched.

Not only did I love working with Greg in the surgery, but he was terrific around the farm as well, and we often worked together on all the jobs that had to be done. He would throw himself body and soul into whatever we were doing. One day, though, when we were digging out a blocked drain, I could sense that he was slacking. He had gone down to town the evening before to, yet again, juggle the impressively large stable of women he ran, and I suspect that he hadn't had much sleep.

"Come on, you randy pillock," I yelled. "You might have shagged yourself to a standstill last night, but there's still work to be done here."

"You're just jealous," he replied with his pantomime villain accent. "You just want to take out your Helen frustrations by squeezing blood from a poor little Polish stone," he added and then accidentally hit himself in the face with the handle of his shovel and set off a spectacular nosebleed that took ages to settle.

While Greg pinched his nose to stem the flow, we took time out from the digging and rested on the bank above the drain.

"You're probably right," I said.

"Well, do something about it," he replied.

I lay back on the wet earth and looked up at the sky. I often spoke to Helen on the phone, of course, but Ginny remained desperately ill, and it looked as if it would be a long time before Helen would be able to come back.

"I'd love to," I said dreamily. "But like what?"

"Like buy a ticket and fly to France," he continued as if stating the obvious.

Evenings with Greg were every bit as enjoyable as those I had spent with his predecessor. Greg wasn't quite in the same kitchen class as Archie, but what he gave away in quality, he more than made up for in quantity. With Greg in charge, I have never eaten so much cabbage in my life and had to excuse myself to patients for weeks after he left.

As it was wintertime during Greg's stay, we spent most of our evenings together in front of the fire rather than out by the lake. One night, Greg turned to me and said, "Paul, I would like your help on a personal matter."

"Delighted to be of assistance," I replied, thinking we were about to have another session disentangling his love life. "Fire away."

"I'd like you to help me choose a name," he said.

"A name for what?"

"For me."

"But you've already got a name," I replied.

"Yes, but while it might have worked in Poland, it doesn't work here. I have decided to change it."

"It's your choice, of course," I said, "but personally I don't see what's wrong with Czczyz. I rather like it. I think it has a certain panache."

We went around the house and gathered up all the dictionaries with lists of names in the back. Then with our research material gathered together, we filled our glasses, settled by the fire, and got down to it.

There were thousands of names to sift through, and we were at it until late. *Smiths*, *Browns*, and *Joneses* were dismissed early as being too ordinary while *Singhs*, *Patels*, and *Nguyens* were discarded as not quite what we were looking for. After a while, Greg came up with the idea that he would like to stay with the same initial, and that simplified things considerably. It was around midnight that he found what he was looking for.

"Eureka!" he shouted excitedly and held up the page for me to see.

"'Cobbledick!'" I said in surprise when I saw what he was pointing at.

"Exactly," he said, "I think it has a nice English sound to it, don't you?"

"You don't feel it might make you sound just a little like a urologist?" I asked, but his mind was already made up.

Initially, everyone else was a little surprised by Greg's choice of name, but then it caught on like wildfire, and at least everyone knew how to say it.

"And is it spelt as one would imagine?" Heather asked in her usual prim way.

"It certainly is," Greg replied. "Just *cobble* and then *dick*."

There was the slightest of pauses. "Right," she said and then after a further pause she said, "Right" again.

▪ ▪ ▪

As we came to the end of his stay, Cobbledick and I decided that we would spend our last weekend together playing golf up on the river courses. I have no idea why we decided on a golfing trip, seeing that I barely know which end of a club to hold and he had never played before, but once we got the idea in our heads, it seemed as if it was the only thing that we could possibly do.

We managed to talk the practice over at Cowley into looking after any emergencies that might present over the weekend, left Heather in charge of the telephone, told her not to employ anyone called Geoffrey, packed our bags, headed north, and had a terrific time.

Hacking our way round those manicured Murray courses during the day, and spending evenings toasting a succession of sunsets with a variety of colored liquids at a number of riverside locations was a lovely way to wrap up the time that we'd spent together. And the golf was good too for, despite Greg's inexperience, it turned out to be a surprisingly tight contest.

My main memories, however, are not of the cut and thrust of the scorecards but rather of his interminable and seemingly pointless Polish jokes, which clearly lost much in translation. I remember one in particular, something to do with Mongolians living in a tent, which he started as we teed off and didn't finish telling until we were nearly back in the clubhouse.

The standout image, however, is none of that. Rather, it is of the final hole we played in front of a packed clubhouse at Yarrawonga. It was a prolonged ordeal, and by the time we had finished chipping backward and forward from bunker to bunker across the green, before finally holing out, we had held up play as far back as the fourteenth fairway.

As we were walking off the green, I happened to glance up at the clubhouse gallery. There was a throng of assembled members on the balcony who had obviously been following our progress with interest and whose numbers had increased markedly during the course of our struggle. At the thought of facing them, I turned bright red.

"Just remember," Greg said when he saw where I was looking, "what other people think of you is none of your business."

"Yes, I know," I replied, "but why don't we go and have a drink somewhere else anyway. It's been a great few weeks," I said to Greg a little while later as we supped at a nearby watering hole.

"It certainly has," he replied. We touched glasses and vowed never to lose contact, and we never have.

▪ ▪ ▪

I phoned Ewa the very next day after receiving her package. Unfortunately, I wasn't able to speak to her in person, so I left a message inviting her to come to Dixon's Bridge the following weekend and have a look around. Two days later, I received a letter.

> My great Carter
>
> I write for to explain you some personal details.
> I am 36 old years.
>
> In Krakow I am pediatrician. It was great fully
> to know I can work in your house.
>
> I will journey on train and deposit Stoney Creek
> 9.32 Satday.

> I have a long blonde hair. My tall is 1.75m. Slim, I shall go with a white dress. More easier to recourse me I shall wear in my left hand a red roses.
>
> Hopping to see you soon, I said you hello from Ewa Kozlowski

Accordingly, and with some excitement, I made my way to the station the following Saturday, pulling into the parking area just as the train was coming to a stop.

Ewa presented herself exactly as she had described, but she needn't have worried about being recognized. Maybe things are different in Krakow Central Railway Station, but at Stoney Creek on a Saturday morning, there is no crowd at all. As the train pulled away, she was the only passenger left standing on the platform, except, that is, for the small boy holding her hand.

We made our greetings, got into the pickup, and headed back to the farm. "This your car?" she asked after a minute or two.

"Yes."

"This doctor's car?" she asked again.

"A *country* doctor's car," I replied.

"Thought maybe Jaguar," she continued.

"Yes, I've often thought Jaguar myself," I replied a little defensively.

Back at the farm, Andre, the small boy, and Nel fell in love at first sight and headed off for some stick throwing while I made some tea.

As it was brewing, I put the roses in a vase, and Ewa had a look around as I hastily cleared some dirty crockery off the table and stowed some washing out of sight.

"No woman lives here?" she asked.

"No, but how…?" I asked.

"Just know these things." She smiled back at me.

"Would you like something to eat?" I asked.

"Love chocolate," she replied, so I got out the Tim Tams.

As we drank our tea and crunched on the chocolate biscuits, I gazed across the kitchen table at her. The sunlight coming in through the window fell across her face and hair. I drew in a sharp breath for she was quite beautiful.

With her chiseled looks, her hourglass figure, and her long blond curls, she looked just like every eastern European femme fatale who has ever appeared in any James Bond movie. And perhaps I am not the only one to think so. When a computer deep in the bowels of the Health Department did eventually decide that Dixon's Bridge was an area of need, and it was therefore appropriate to sign off on the paperwork needed for Ewa to practice there, she officially became Dr. AK 47-007.

"Are you married?" I asked.

"No."

"Boyfriend?"

"No," she said again, "but why you ask?"

"No reason," I said. "Just making conversation."

As we sat there, chatting in the sunshine, I learned how she had come to be sitting at my kitchen table.

With Ewa tied up doing endless hours of hospital work back in Krakow, her husband had felt in need of company. Coming home early one day because of a power cut, Ewa had walked in on a scene she wasn't supposed to have seen and had made her views of what she thought about it all crystal clear by attacking the soft and fleshier parts of the disturbed lovers with her high-heeled shoes.

Recognizing that she needed time out, and keen to protect the husband, who was their senior surgeon, Ewa's hospital recommended her for the job of looking after a group of children with leukemia who were being sent for a holiday in Australia. Ewa not only enjoyed having the break, but she also liked what she saw down under and, on her return to Poland, immediately made plans to come back.

Just two years after her first visit, and with a visa hot off the press, Ewa picked Andre up from school one afternoon, said goodbye to her mother, caught a taxi to the airport, and left.

Back in Australia, and like Tamas before her, Ewa was disappointed to find that the qualifications that had entitled her to work in a prestigious teaching hospital back home counted for nothing on the other side of the globe. After getting over her initial disappointment, however, she simply got herself a job as a hospital cleaner, and then rolled up her sleeves and spent her evenings studying for the Australian examinations. She passed with flying colors at her first attempt and had been working in the emergency department of a small country hospital in the back blocks of New South Wales ever since.

"Why move to Dixon's Bridge?" I asked.

"Like Melbourne," she replied.

"And would you like me to offer you a job right now, or would you prefer me to wait until after I have shown you around?" I asked when she finished her tea.

"Only afterwards," she replied. "Like suspense."

I drove Ewa and Andre over to the practice and then around the district, ending up at Heather and Rob's for lunch. Heather was her usual friendly self, but Rob, whose eyes were out on stalks the whole mealtime, hardly said a word.

"She might be very nice," Heather confided in me as we were leaving, "but I do know one thing for sure—Rob won't be going along to her with any of his medical problems. And you better mind your P's and Q's as well, young man," she turned at me and said.

"I've no idea what you're talking about," I replied innocently.

"I think you do."

"Are you suggesting that impure thoughts might have crossed my mind?" I asked incredulously. "Because if so, you couldn't be further from the mark."

"Scratch a man, you find a man," she replied darkly.

"Well," I said when Ewa and I got back to the farm, "what did you think of the practice?"

"Very nice," she replied.

"And would you like a job?" I asked cautiously.

"Yes," she said, "but there is condition I must insist on."

"And what is that?" I asked a little apprehensively.

"Must have purple room."

"Consider it done," I said, smiling with relief.

▪ ▪ ▪

Back at Woongarra, after an evening meal of coq au vin, we sat and chatted until late. When it was finally time to go to bed, despite the reassurances I had given Heather earlier, I admit to giving Ewa the old nod, nod, wink, wink.

"What are you doing with your face?" she asked.

"Giving you an invitation," I replied.

"Never mix sex and partnership," she said as she wagged her finger.

"Partnership?" I asked in surprise.

"Isn't that what you are offering me?"

"Well, I suppose it was, in a way," I answered lamely.

"Well, that's that then," she said decisively, and we went our separate ways.

▪ ▪ ▪

Like Greg before her, Ewa was an immediate success in the practice. Within weeks, she had her own following and had taken over the lioness's share of all the girlie stuff.

"I feel safe going out to dinner parties again," I told people.

The language barrier wasn't much of a problem either. Not only did Ewa's English improve rapidly, but unlike Greg, she didn't speak as if she were trying to cough up a frog at the same time.

Spelling she found more difficult, and she still occasionally produces howlers. Only recently, I came across some notes of hers where she'd recorded that some poor fellow was having a problem with his *testickles.*

As soon as it could be arranged, Ewa and Andre moved from Woongarra into a house out on Five Rocks Road. And to get her mobile, I borrowed the old Datsun Bluebird that had been sitting in one of Trevor's sheds for years.

"What is this?" Ewa said, turning up her nose when she first saw it.

"It's a Mercedes," I said. "One of their early models."

She looked at me with a frown for a few moments, and then her face relaxed.

"Good." She chuckled. "Always wanted a Mercedes. Will write and let my mother know."

Ewa took to Dixon's Bridge like a duck to water and, these days, is even married to a local fellow. He is a nice man who makes her laugh and who she is extremely unlikely to have to attack with her shoes. She is highly experienced these days but, even so, still occasionally finds Australian country practice different from anything she experienced in Poland.

"Paul, we have some unusual patients," she recently said with a shake of her head over our morning tea.

"How do you mean?" I asked, and she went on to mention the name of a delightful elderly couple who live on a small farmlet over toward Heddington.

"The husband came in for a prostate test," Ewa said, eyes wide open. "And, Paul, guess what I found."

"Or didn't find," I replied knowingly.

"*Exactly*," Ewa agreed passionately, "or didn't find. No prostate, no penis, no scrotum, no nothing. Just vagina."

"And what did you do? I asked, intrigued as to how she had handled the situation.

"Well, I was about to say, 'Hello, what's going on here?' but then I stopped and didn't say a thing. I just got him to sit up and get dressed again. I told him that everything was fine and then said that I'd like see him again in a year's time."

"Good girl," I applauded. "You have come a long way."

RECIPES FOR DISASTER

Tim Tams

Always keep well stocked.

20

JULES

Late one afternoon, an elegant, well-dressed woman of about my own age came in for an appointment. She was new to the practice.

"Paul," I introduced myself as we shook hands. "I don't think we've met before."

"Jules," she said in a lovely English accent that was cultured but not affected. "I don't think we have either. But then perhaps it's not surprising as I only arrived in Australia a week ago."

"And are you here on a holiday?" I asked.

"No," she said with the faintest hint of a blush. "I'm here to get married."

"How wonderful," I said, and in answer to my further questioning, she informed me that the lucky man was Harry. "Ah, so *you're* Jules," I added, for I knew Harry quite well.

Many years before, there had been a move to locate a rifle range in the Mullaways, and it had been Harry who had mobilized the forces against it. We had met once or twice in the surgery, and he inveigled me onto his committee as a medical expert when he heard that I'd seen a few gunshot wounds. After the plan for the range eventually sank under the weight of the protest orchestrated by Harry, we remained friends. We didn't live in one another's pockets, but we caught up now and again. It was on one of those occasions that he told me about Jules.

"I understand you met him at university," I said to her.

"Yes," she replied, "a very long time ago."

"So I understand," I said. "And now, since we seem to have your social life sorted out, I wonder how I can be of help."

"Nothing much," she said. "I just need something for my tummy. It's probably the change of water or jet lag, but for the last few days, I've had a bit of an upset."

"Not a problem," I replied and asked her to hop onto the couch so that I could check things over.

When I finished my examination, I sat facing her across the desk. "Jules," I said, "I don't think you have a tummy upset, and I don't think it's a matter of just giving you something for it."

"Oh dear," she said, "you're sounding rather serious."

"Yes, I'm afraid I am," I replied. "You're much paler than you have any right to be, and there's a large lump in your tummy that shouldn't be there.

"Oh," she said. "Well, I'm pretty sure I'm not pregnant, so what else could it be?"

"Any number of things," I replied, "but it *is* just possible that it's something unpleasant. Well, you did ask," I added in answer to her startled look, "and I've always been a rotten liar."

"Yes. Yes, thank you," she replied, "and now at least I know why you were looking serious."

I organized some tests and scans, made sure she was spending the evening with Harry, and arranged to meet her again when we had the results.

I'm not sure that I've ever given worse news to someone that I've just met for the first time, and after she left, I felt very flat.

Heather came in with a cup of tea. "Are you okay?" she asked.

"So-so," I said and then reflected that at least the modern openness was infinitely preferable to how things had been between doctors and patients when I first qualified.

"What operation have you had?" I remember asking a patient when I was new to the wards.

"You'd have to ask the surgeon that," he had replied.

"So what made him perform it?"

"You'd have to ask him that as well."

"But why are you in hospital?"

"I've no idea. Surely *you* should know. You're the doctor."

I'd like to be able to say that I had then asked the man what had brought him to the hospital, and he'd replied "an ambulance," but I didn't and he didn't, so I can't.

Harry had attended the practice long before I joined Felix. I understand that he was always a serious and studious young man and, in his last year at school, had come to the surgery with a carefully written list of medical concerns. Felix had examined him, run a few tests, and then written him a prescription for a hearty diet, a regular walk with the family dog, and a hobby to take his mind off his health.

It must have been the right advice, for Harry not only finished his final year but went on to became the very first member ever of his family to go to a university. Aware that he was the family flag bearer, Harry determined to make the most of his new opportunity and spent much more of his time in the library and much less time at parties than many of his fellows.

On the occasion of his graduation, Harry's parents traveled to Melbourne for only the second time in their life. It was a day of great rejoicing, for Harry had not only topped his year but also secured a scholarship to Oxford University.

On one of our evenings together, out at his place, Harry stoked up the fire after we had eaten and then poured each of us a scotch. Not normally a man to talk about himself, for some reason, he chose that evening to reminisce, and it was late indeed before I found my way home.

He started by telling me how much he'd enjoyed his time at Oxford and talked nostalgically about the Bodleian Library, the quads, and the bumps rowing races. He also added that he hadn't felt homesick as his mother had regularly sent over food parcels loaded up with all his favorites.

He did well academically, he said, and after his graduation was invited to stay on for a further year as part of the teaching staff. It was at the orientation meeting for new teachers that he first saw Jules.

"I only met her because of that extra year," he said. "I often think how easily our paths might never have crossed."

Harry said that Jules had caught his eye from the very beginning. He didn't get to speak to her that first day, however, as she had been constantly surrounded by a crowd of admirers. Harry said he couldn't believe his luck when the dean later asked him if she could share his study.

"And love blossomed instantly?" I asked, but Harry shook his head.

"No, not at all," he said. "Firstly, we were both extremely busy with our research and teaching commitments and then there was my damn shyness."

"As the weeks passed by, though, things changed," Harry said, and it seemed that two young people spending endless hours in close proximity eventually did its usual magic. By the end of the first term, they were lovers.

"It was a wonderful time," Harry said, gazing dreamily into the fire, "and then one evening, when we were curled up on the sofa, taking an evening off from our work, she quietly said, 'Harry, there's something I have to tell you, and you're not going to like it.'

"I looked down at her head resting on my shoulder, and I could feel her heart beating against me," he continued, "and I said, 'Well, in that case, perhaps I don't want to hear it.' She was quiet for a while and then said, 'Perhaps you're right' and got up and made some tea."

Harry said that he really enjoyed his teaching post, but it seemed to come to an end all in a rush. Suddenly, he realized that he had known Jules for almost a year.

"I felt we should recognize the event," he said, "and even got her a present."

At Jules's suggestion, they dined in to celebrate their first circuit round the sun together, and after they had finished their meal, they sat and held hands across the table.

"You are the love of my life," Harry said.

"I didn't know you cared." I smiled back at him.

"Not you, you silly sod. That's what I said to her," he said and got up and poked some life back into the fire. "And then she told me that I was the love of hers."

"I then told her that I would shortly be going back to Australia and asked if she would do me the honor of coming with me as my wife. I was about to get out the ring that I'd bought," he continued, "when I realized that she'd gone very quiet.

"'I'm afraid I can't,' she whispered, 'I'm already married.'"

"I bet that got your attention," I said.

"It certainly did," Harry replied. "Anyway, there was a long silence, and then I asked her if she would like to expand a little on what she'd just said.

"Apparently, she was married to a guy called Brendan," Harry said. "She'd been an undergraduate at the time and had met him at a Vietnam rally in Grosvenor Square. He was a senior lecturer at her college, and she attended some of his classes. He had burnt an effigy of Uncle Sam, and she had married him the next day.

"I understand that, at least to start with, things had gone okay, but that one day, she had walked unannounced into his office and found one of her friends sprawled across the desk with Brendan on top of her. Apparently, Jules had then put up with an entire passing parade, but the final straw was when she caught him back at their flat with a couple of overseas first years.

"The university hushed everything up by sending Brendan off to UCLA, and Jules said that she hadn't heard from him since, until just recently when he'd contacted her and told her that he was coming back to England.

"I asked Jules to come away with me anyway," Harry said, "but she said that she couldn't and that she had to stay and sort out the mess. I begged her to change her mind, but she wouldn't."

After we made ourselves some coffee, Harry continued.

"Three weeks later, I caught a flight back home, and I've been here ever since," he said, gesturing at the house around him. "And apart from the year with Pippa, I've spent all that time on my own."

"Yes, well, I'm beginning to know how that feels," I said as I got up and stretched.

▪ ▪ ▪

A few days after her first visit, Jules came in to discuss the results of her tests.

"Well, I've got some good news, and I've got some bad news," I said as she sat down. "The good news is that we know exactly what the problem is, and the bad news is that it's not good news," I added and then went on to tell her about her cancer.

I phoned a hospital that specialized in the sort of help Jules required, and they were very cooperative, right up to the time when I told them that she was from overseas.

"So she's not covered under Medicare?" they asked.

"No, I'm afraid that she isn't," I replied.

"What did they say?" Jules asked when I put the phone down.

"They suggested that you get on the next flight home and get all your treatment back in the UK," I replied.

"I am not going back," she said calmly. "I am going to stay here with my fiancé. I've waited a long time to come here to get married, and that is what I'm going to do."

Over the next few days, there was a flurry of phone calls to various government departments to see if there was any way that Jules could be treated locally. Whoever we spoke to was invariably polite, but the responses we got all sounded like something out of a *Yes, Minister* script. For a week or so, it seemed as if Jules really might have to pack her bags and go home.

Then just a day or so later, Jules got a call from the Department of Busybodying. They told her that after full consideration of all aspects of her case and in cognizance of the current reciprocal arrangements that existed between Australia and the United Kingdom, it had been decided that, on this occasion, and without setting any precedents, it was considered appropriate to allow an exemption under section H, paragraph four, subsection 23 of the act passed in 1986, being in full compliance with amendment 271 tabled in 1998.

Jules immediately phoned the surgery and let me know. "And what on earth does that all mean?" I asked.

"That I can stay," she replied.

"Well, why didn't they just say that?" I asked again.

"It's against their interests," she said. "They get paid by the word."

When Jules visited the surgery the following day, I was able to tell her that I'd heard that the hospital had given the green light, a surgeon had been organized for her operation, and a date had been set.

"Thank you so much," she replied and then asked for the address.

"Surely you're not planning to get there under your own steam?" I asked.

"Of course," she said. "Harry's had to go interstate, and I don't have any ambulance cover. Don't worry," she continued as she jangled a set of ignition keys, "I can look after myself."

Meaghan wrote down the address of the hospital, and then she and Heather and I stood by the front door of the surgery and watched as Jules disappeared noisily, but as elegantly as ever, down the high street on a Harley Roadster.

"Now that," Meaghan said as the bike eventually disappeared from view, "is what I call classy."

■ ■ ■

Back in Australia, Harry didn't get over his disappointment at losing Jules. One day, when he was feeling especially low, he came into the surgery looking for help, and it was then that, as a recent arrival to the countryside, I met him for the first time. He didn't want anything in the way of medication. I think he just wanted a bit of a chat.

"Keep yourself really busy," I advised when he finished.

"Yes," he replied dully, "Felix already told me to do that."

Over the months that followed, while Harry didn't resolve his loneliness, he took my advice and distracted himself from it with his work at the university. He threw himself into every research project he could find and took on every possible teaching commitment.

Then a year or so after his return, and seemingly on the spur of the moment, he married Pippa, who he'd just met at a friend's fortieth. The wedding was in South Australia, where her parents lived, and I was delighted to get an invite.

It was a memorable event for a number of reasons—the first being that the bride came up the aisle on a camel, and the second was the table on which I found myself sitting at the reception.

I'm not sure who had been in charge of the seating arrangements, but they had shown a breathtaking recklessness in arranging table number one. Apart from myself, there was the bride's father with his pretty new wife and the bride's stepfather with his new fiancée. There was an old lover of the bride's mother who thought it very funny to keep asking if anyone could still smell camel, and then there was the bride's mother, together with her nineteen-year-old Turkish-speaking boyfriend. Shortly after the soup, she winked at me from behind her boyfriend's back, and as she did so, it occurred to me that I was the only man at the table who didn't *know* her, in the Old Testament sense.

The marriage lasted just a little over a year. Even that was a surprise, for I'm not sure that either of them really knew what had glued their relationship together in the first place. While Harry preferred walking in the Mullaways, Pippa liked to party, party, party.

There was no great explosion. The relationship just fizzled out, and they went their separate ways. Pippa went back to Melbourne, and Harry stayed on with farming and academia.

▪ ▪ ▪

For the next twenty years, Harry focused his energies on his research, on writing learned articles, and on climbing ever higher up the academic ladder. Eventually, he was given a chair. When he won an award for a series of papers he wrote on geothermal warming, he was invited to address a conference in Montreal as the keynote speaker.

I didn't see Harry for a while, but then I bumped into him while having a coffee one Saturday morning in the new café down near the bridge. Harry came over as soon as he saw me and sat down. "You don't mind if I join you?" he asked.

"Delighted," I assured him. "You're looking very pleased with yourself. Things obviously went well in Canada."

"Dreadful, actually," he said with a smile.

"Well then, you don't look in the least upset about it," I replied.

"I'm not," he continued. "As you know, I went over there to give a lecture. It was a very big do indeed. When the time came for my presentation, I was duly introduced, warmly welcomed, and then got started. I'd been going for about ten minutes or so, and I was really working up a good head of steam, when I caught sight of Jules in the audience.

"I didn't have to look twice. I instantly knew it was her and stopped dead in my tracks. It hadn't even crossed my mind that she would be there.

"My head was in such a spin that I could hardly think what I was saying. I eventually fumbled through the rest of my presentation, but I couldn't concentrate on anything and made a complete mess of question time."

"Did you speak to her?" I asked.

"Well, what do you think," he replied. "As soon as I got off the stage, I skipped an official cocktail party and went looking for her. It took me a while, but I eventually caught up with her, and we finished up having dinner. But the best bit," he continued, looking like a cat that has swallowed the cream, "is that we're going to get married."

"That's fantastic," I said, "but I thought you said she already had a husband?"

"She did," he said, "but she doesn't now. Brendan did come back from America, but apparently it was simply to show off his new girlfriend and organize a divorce."

"And how did the conversation get around to marriage?" I asked.

"Easy." He laughed. "When I heard what had happened, I proposed on the spot." Harry looked happier than I had ever seen him.

"You look great," I said.

"Well, she's my soul mate," he replied.

"How can you be so sure about things like that?" I asked.

"Good question," he said. "Perhaps it's just that I have never felt as good as when I'm with her," and I knew exactly how he felt.

"Will I get an invite?" I asked when he got back from getting more coffees. "After all, I came to your last one."

"You certainly will," he replied.

"In that case," I said, "I have one small request."

"And what's that?"

"That this time I get to choose my own table," I said, but in the end, it wasn't necessary.

▪ ▪ ▪

Over the years, I have been lucky enough to be invited to weddings in all sorts of interesting places. They have ranged from cathedrals to aboriginal meeting places, from bandstands to old-growth forests, and from sailing clubs to pubs. They have all been lovely occasions, but if I had to pick a favorite single moment from all of them, it would be when Pol and Mitch got hitched in the public bar at the Whistle Stop. When the time came for Pol to pledge herself, her nerves failed her, and she called a halt the proceedings.

"This is the fucking scariest thing I've ever done, you know," she announced to the assembled crowd and then, together with the rest of the bridal party, fortified herself with a stiff drink and a fag before going on to eventually, and rather breathlessly, say "I do."

Despite all this, until Harry's telephone call a couple of days later, I had never before been invited to a wedding in a hospital.

Harry and Jules had originally planned to get married out on the farm after she recovered from her operation. The arrangements were brought forward, however, when things didn't go according to plan. The cancer had been far more widespread than expected, and the operation had taken much longer. Jules had lost a huge amount of blood during the procedure and had finished up in intensive care.

Just for once, I was early for something, and arrived at the hospital before everyone else. Jules had been put in a side ward for the occasion. She was looking pale and ill.

"You look nice," I said, for the nurses had made a garland for her hair. "I love the dress," I added, nodding at the standard hospital issue. "Blue suits you."

"I had it brought up from the linen department specially"—she smiled weakly up at me—"together with the fashion accessories." She waved a hand at all the plastic tubing.

We sat for a few moments in silence.

"Jules," I said, "it's not really my place, but before the others arrive, do you mind if I ask you a question about something?"

"Not at all," she said.

"Well, Harry told me that you got divorced pretty much as soon as Brendan got back from America. Did you ever think of letting Harry know?"

"Of course," she said quietly to my astonishment. "I flew out to Australia as soon as the papers came through. I wanted it to be a surprise, so I didn't let him know that I was coming.

"I was so excited when I landed and took a taxi straight from the airport to the farm. When I arrived there, I was greeted by a woman who was sitting in a swinging seat on the porch. I asked her if Harry was at home. She said no, he wasn't there, but that since she was his wife, I could leave any messages with her. I was stunned. It had never even occurred to me. I made some feeble excuse or other about being there and then caught the same taxi back to town. I think that the flight back to England was the longest I've ever had."

"Goodness," I said, "I can imagine."

"Can you?" she asked gently. "Harry's been the only man I ever loved. The only one with whom I've ever felt complete. I wonder," she continued quietly after a pause, "can you really imagine that?"

"Well, as a matter of fact, I can," I said and went on to tell her about a woman on the other side of the world, the very thought of whom drove me wild with desire.

"So how does that work?" Jules asked. "With the distance, I mean."

"It doesn't," I replied sadly. "I'm hoping against hope that she'll be coming home soon."

We sat for a few moments in silence, and this time it was Jules who broke the silence.

"This is supposed to be a cheerful day, and we both seem a bit flat," she said. "So before the others get here, why don't you cheer me up with one of the stories Harry says you're so good at?"

I thought blankly for a moment and was about to admit defeat when something suddenly occurred to me.

"Don't think," I said to her, "that you're the first person I've ever seen in a hospital bed wearing a wedding dress, because you're not. When I was a medical student, doing my obstetric posting, a very pretty redhead, accompanied by her pale and freckly new husband, was brought into the labor ward wearing what I believe is known in the trade as a meringue.

"Apparently, the happy couple had just finished signing the registry book when the young lady interrupted proceedings by breaking her waters. She was pretty far advanced by the time she reached us, and we didn't even have time to take her dress off.

"Despite the meringue, however, the labor went smoothly, and the only thing of note in the entire proceedings came when she produced a beautiful coal-black baby.

"There was a stunned silence in the labor suite for a while, and then the redhead looked up at us all and said, 'Funnily enough, the thought had crossed my mind.'

"'Well sod you,' the husband had angrily replied and had then got up and stormed out, never to be seen again."

"I never know whether to believe your stories or not." Jules chuckled quietly.

I was still imploring Jules to believe in me when the door to the cubicle flew open, and Harry and two of his university colleagues burst in, singing that well-known theme from *Lohengrin.*

"Hello, hello, hello," they stopped in their tracks and said. "Looks like we're just in the nick of time to prevent some monkey business in the bridal chamber."

Jules and I were in the process of protesting our innocence when the door opened again. This time it was the hospital padre who fussed over everyone, made sure Harry's friends had remembered the rings, and generally got us all organized.

Two days later, I saw Harry in the coffee shop again, and this time it was me who went over to join him. He looked terrible as he glanced silently up at me.

"How are you?" I said as I sat down and put an arm round his shoulders.

"How do you reckon," he replied.

"Yes, stupid question," I said, and Harry didn't have to say anything else for I'd already been contacted by the hospital.

The day after the wedding, Jules had collapsed with another bleed in her tummy. She was taken back to the theater, but they weren't able to stop the flow. An entire team had worked on her for hours, but despite every effort, Jules had eventually floated quietly and elegantly away from this world.

"Sorry to hear about Jules," Heather said to me later on in the day.

"Thanks," I replied flatly. "Perhaps the trick is to get everything important done right now and not just wait for things to happen on their own."

"Well, we've all been telling you that for ages," she replied, "and *you* could start by stopping messing about and going and actually doing what you've been saying you want to do."

After the afternoon surgery, I was idly sifting through the huge pile of correspondence that magically appears on my desk on a daily basis when I came across a letter with a French stamp on it. I pushed everything else aside and opened it up. I imagined that it would be one of Helen's usual bright and breezy missives that brighten up my day, but it wasn't that at all. She wrote to tell me that Ginny had passed away, that her brother was not showing the slightest interest in his responsibilities as a father, and that as a result, she felt obliged to stay on in Paris for at least a while longer to continue looking after the children.

I leaned over and pressed the buzzer on the phone.

"Heather," I said, "could you please get me on the next possible flight to Paris," and I heard her swear for the very first time.

"About bloody time," she replied.

21

HELEN

Helen's letter telling me she had decided to stay on in Paris to look after the girls galvanized me into action. It now seemed that there was every likelihood of Helen slipping out of my life forever, which I absolutely did not want to happen.

Off and on, over the last couple of years, I had dreamed about going over to France, and plenty of people had certainly encouraged me to do so. For a variety of lame excuses, however, apart from getting myself a passport, I had done nothing about it. Jules's death changed everything.

Ewa said that she was happy to look after the practice while I was away, the people at the travel agency made all the necessary arrangements, and many of my regulars wished me well for my adventure. One or two of them even bade me "bon voyage."

I decided not to tell Helen that I was coming, for despite how things had turned out for Jules, I still wanted my arrival to be a surprise. As the plane hurtled down the runway and the wheels left the ground, I could think of nothing but success. After all, I was going to meet my soul mate.

"Any special reason for the trip?" the hostess had asked.

"There certainly is," I replied, "I'm going to see the love of my life."

"Well, that's wonderful." She smiled and asked if I'd like a glass of champagne.

It was only once we were in the stratosphere that doubts began to creep into my mind. Would the trip turn out well, or would it all turn to tears? Would Helen be pleased to see me, or would fate intervene and prevent our paths from even crossing? Perhaps I was stupid not to have let her know I was coming. Perhaps she already had found somebody else.

And as I fitfully dozed, the negatives kept circling around inside my head. Would she even still like me? Would she even want to see me?

I had, of course, told her that I'd been unwell. She had sounded very concerned over the phone at the time and had written me some lovely letters since, but perhaps she was just being polite and was hiding her real feelings. Perhaps she really thought how lucky she had been to escape. Just for once, I realized that what someone else thought of me really *was* my business.

In regard to the wisdom of actually making the journey, however, I never had any doubts at all. Whatever trip wires and snares might lie ahead, I was doggedly determined to face them. Alex's advice, given all that time before, was my guiding light, and there was no possibility of even thinking of turning back.

"Well, shut up and take a bloody risk then," I could hear her saying, and here I was.

After all, I had never felt as good as when I had been with Helen. Like Alex with Rhonda, like Jules with Harry, I had never felt as complete as when in Helen's company. She might have started out as a teenage infatuation, but she was now a great deal more than that. She was now the other half of my adult soul. I turned to share all this with the person in the seat next to me, with whom I had been chatting earlier, but she had fallen asleep and was snoring.

Later, in a darkened cabin and watching some totally forgettable film on a four-inch screen, I had another thought: would Helen even recognize me? I pulled out my passport and looked at the picture. It wasn't a pretty sight. I certainly didn't look at all well when the photo had been taken and could only hope that I had improved a bit since.

I am still a poor sleeper at the best of times, and overnight plane trips are no exception. As we continued to rumble through the night, I hardly so much as closed my eyes. Instead, I did some stretching exercises, made a mess of an 'easy' Sudoku, failed miserably on a general knowledge quiz, and then got up and walked up and down the cabin for a while.

Somewhere, high over India, and tidying up the stretch pouch in front of me, I came across the card that Heather and Meaghan had given me as I was leaving. It was a picture of a frog fighting desperately to avoid being swallowed by a heron. "Whatever happens," it said, "never, ever give in," and I wholeheartedly agreed.

The card reminded me of something that had happened just a week or so before leaving. I had been on my way to the Base Hospital for an afternoon's workshop on the latest in prostate care. The freeway that leads there runs through some fairly deserted country, and in the middle of nowhere, I'd had a puncture and been forced to pull over.

After doing the necessary repairs, I was in the process of stowing everything back in the trunk when I happened to glance up. There, only a few yards from where I was parked, on the other side of the final remains of what had once been a farm fence, was a large, dilapidated wooden sign that said, "*ROCKS FOR SALE.*"

Where I had been forced to stop is not a pretty spot. The country there is full of thistles and rocks and gives the impression that whatever damage hasn't resulted from nature itself, has certainly been finished off by mankind. Farming out there must be hard indeed, and the abandoned houses scattered over the hills seem proof that there have been many lean years between the fat ones.

About a hundred yards or so behind "*ROCKS FOR SALE,*" there was a low cluster of forlorn-looking structures that were leaning on one another in what appeared to be a last desperate bid to defy gravity. They were clearly inhabited, however, for there was washing on the line.

I imagined that whoever lived there had taken to rock selling during the leaner years when all else had failed. I have no idea how successful the new venture had proven to be, but if it had paid all the bills, then I guess there would have been no need to erect the other three signs that stood nearby, each one younger by some years than its predecessor.

The second sign said, "*VEHICLES NEW AND USED.*" There must have been a time when the highway was much smaller than it is now and traffic traveled more slowly. Maybe this place was even a welcome break in the journey, and when travelers stopped for a while, vehicles may well have been discussed, but that is all long gone. Today the homestead might as well be a hundred miles from the road as a hundred yards, for the highway now comprises six lanes of traffic, three of them racing from A to B, with the other three just as keen to get from B to A.

Into the third sign, "*FULL BODY MASSAGE,*" the passersby can read whatever they choose. Maybe it means exactly what it says, but then again maybe it means something entirely different. I have no means of knowing; but one thing is sure, if you *did* decide to treat yourself to a full body massage, then it might be best to park your car out the back—unless, that is, you want ten thousand people on their way to A and a further ten thousand on their way to B knowing that in approximately half an hour's time, you'll be as loose as a goose.

The youngest sign, "*AFRICAN LION SAFARIS,*" was painted on the side of an old shipping container

"How did the meeting go?" Meaghan asked me the next morning back at the surgery.

"Great," I replied.

"Learn anything interesting?" she asked. "I certainly did," I replied.

"Well?" she asked again.

"That in the lean years, if rocks don't sell and no one wants a car, just break out the massage oil and get in a few lions."

▪ ▪ ▪

When I got off the plane in Paris, it was five o'clock in the morning. I had the worst French food I have ever tasted in the airport cafeteria, mucked about until seven, and then caught a taxi out to Helen's address. I spent the journey drinking in the iconic scenery and listening to the Somali taxi driver talk about his son who was in medical school in Boston.

The address wasn't in a part of town my driver knew well, but we eventually found our destination. Together with my bags, I was deposited on the footpath, and the taxi drove away. I stood still for a few moments as I looked around, took three slow deep breaths, then climbed the steps, and with a beating heart, knocked on the door.

There was no answer. More knocking produced the same result and also that sense that there was no one home. I felt more than a little deflated.

I didn't even know which part of Paris I was in, so I decided to just sit on the steps and wait for a bit while I thought things through. I leaned against the railings and having hardly slept a wink on the plane, promptly fell asleep. I was awakened by rain running down the side of my neck, under my collar, and on my chest. I had no idea how long I had been asleep, but when I woke, I was wet through and freezing cold.

I gathered up my luggage and trudged across the road to *Le Paradou*, which looked inviting from the outside and also had the advantage of being warm and dry on the inside. I hung up my dripping coat on the rack, found myself a seat by the window that looked back over to Helen's apartment, and ordered a coffee while I decided what to do next.

When I'd thawed out and dried off, I tried Helen's home and mobile numbers, but neither of them answered. There seemed no point in wandering the streets, so I simply continued to sit there, looking out across the road and ordering more coffee. By lunchtime, Yvette, the lady who ran the place, and I were on first-name terms.

Sometime around midafternoon, Yvette bent toward my ear and confidentially asked me what sort of criminals I was on the lookout for. She knew just about everyone locally, she confided, and perhaps she could be of some help. Initially, she was rather disappointed to learn that I wasn't actually a policeman, but she perked up when I told her that this was, however, a stakeout.

"Pour qui?"[22] she asked.

"Pour une femme fatale," I said with hooded eyes and told her about Helen and the girls. To my pleasant surprise, Yvette knew them well. Apparently, they often popped into the café. Yvette hadn't seen them for a few days, however, but would ask around to see if she could find out where they were. She then went and got me another coffee because, she said, it was important at such times to remain fully alert.

It was at around four o'clock that I suddenly caught sight of Helen walking along on the other side of the street. I shot out of the café and, forgetting that the French drive on the wrong side of the road, nearly got myself killed trying to get across to her. By the time I had extricated myself from the traffic, she was a little way ahead of me, so I called out and ran after her. In just a few seconds, I caught up with her, put a hand on her shoulder, and with a big smile on my face, spun her around.

A woman I had never seen in my life before stared at me in horror as she backed away.

"Que voulez-vous?"[23] she squeaked in fright.

"Pardonnez-moi," I said, turning crimson with embarrassment. "Mon erreur." Same height, same shape, same hairstyle, even the same way of walking. Just a completely different person.

Later, when my nerves had eventually settled down again and the day started changing into night, I found my way to a small nearby hotel that belonged to Yvette's sister. The reception was manned by two tiny pointy-eared bulldogs, and the elevator was a tight fit, even for one, with my luggage having to come up separately.

Next day, back at *Le Paradou*, things went on much the same as they had before, except that I didn't terrify the living daylights out of any passersby. The hours dragged by even more slowly than

---

22. For who?
23. What do you want?

they had the day before, and I had to cut back on the coffee because my hands had started shaking.

Around lunchtime, Yvette came and told me she had found out that Helen and the girls had gone away on a holiday. Nobody knew where they had gone, or for how long, but it was understood that it might be for some time. I unsuccessfully tried Helen's numbers yet again and then sadly decided to call an end to my vigil. Obviously, it had been a mistake not to let Helen know that I was coming.

Yvette asked me if I was going back to Australia, but I reassured her that I was simply taking a break.

"I'll stay in Paris for a few days," I said. "I'll go and look at some galleries and museums and then I'll come back and have another go. There's no way that I'd ever let the heron win," I added, but she didn't understand me.

Yvette organized a taxi and, together with all the regulars, shared a farewell cognac with me while we waited for it to arrive.

As I was finishing my drink, the taxi pulled up. I rather sadly gathered up my things, gave Yvette a peck on the cheek, thanked her for all her help, waved goodbye to the regulars, and went outside. As I opened the taxi door to get in, a woman stepped out.

"Paul?" She looked at me and asked with an expression of complete disbelief.

"Paul?" she asked again when, having temporarily lost the power of speech, I failed to answer.

"Wha…wha…" I replied when I finally found my voice again.

"Paul, it *is* you! What on earth are you doing here?" Helen persisted, standing in front of me. "What a wonderful, wonderful surprise," she said excitedly and threw her arms around me.

She looked stunning. More fully clad but more beautiful than Ayesha by far, and as she stood back, I silently drank her in.

"Well, don't I get a hug as well?" Helen asked, and I obliged in spades.

"Hi," I said when I eventually put her down.

"Is that it?" she replied. "Hi?"

"No, no," I quickly corrected myself and then said all the things that I'd been practicing on the plane. There were quite a lot of them, and it took me quite a while.

It was at this point that two very neat but rather sad-looking children also got out of the taxi. Helen introduced me, and they both solemnly shook me by the hand.

"Bon jour," they said.

"Bon jour, Lucy. Bon jour, Imogen," I replied. "I'm sorry I didn't let you know I was coming," I added, "but I wanted to surprise you."

"Well, you've certainly done that," Helen replied.

"Good," I said, "now please pinch me."

"Say that again," she replied.

"Just pinch me," I repeated, "so that I know you're not simply a dream I'm having."

She obliged, and it hurt, so she obviously wasn't.

"Actually, you're lucky to have caught us," Helen said. "We've been away for a few days, and we weren't due to come back for another week or so. We've only returned now because the hotel accidentally double-booked our room."

"You wouldn't know the name of the clerk responsible for the muck up, would you?" I asked. "Only I wouldn't mind sending them some flowers."

Just then another taxi pulled up, apparently expecting to take someone into town.

"So what on earth are you doing in Paris?" Helen asked after the second taxi had been sorted out. "Is there a medical conference on or something?"

"What?" I replied. "What do you think I'm doing in Paris? I've come here to see you."

"Oh," Helen said quietly.

"There's no one else, is there?" I asked.

"No," she replied with a shake of her head.

"Thank God for that," I continued.

"So what now?" Helen asked.

"Well, having traipsed halfway round the world looking for someone I'm rather fond of, and having finally found her," I replied, "I thought I might like to take her out for dinner tonight."

"Well, that would be lovely." Helen smiled with her whole face. "I had something planned, but I can easily put it off, and I'll arrange a sitter for the girls. Have you organized yourself any accommodation, by the way?" Helen continued, and when I shook my head, she added, "Well, would you like to come and stay with us then?"

"Now let me think about that," I replied with a look of mock surprise.

"Good," she said, "in that case I'll make up the spare bed."

"I don't think..." I started to say and was about to discuss the matter in more detail when I became aware of the children looking at me and decided, just for the moment, to let it go.

▪ ▪ ▪

That night, Helen and I dined on one of the restaurant boats that spend their evenings floating up and down the Seine. They had caught my eye in a magazine back home, and it turned out to be a wonderful choice. The atmosphere was stunning, the string quartet was sublime, the food was to die for, the scenery was the world's most beautiful city, and the company was the world's most ever beautiful woman, with the possible exception of Audrey Hepburn. It was completely and exactly not at all like that evening when Helen had come up to the farm.

"Why don't you try the trout?" I asked as we read the menu, and we both laughed.

"That evening made a big impact on me," she said.

"I bet it did," I said. "And I'm sorry that this just isn't up to the same standard," I added, and we laughed again.

"By the way," Helen said quietly as we were finishing our entrees, "are you well? You certainly look it." And before I could reply, she continued, "I was so sad when I got your news. I felt completely helpless stuck here, on the other side of the world. I really wanted to fly back and be with you, but Ginny was so ill by then that I just couldn't."

"I totally understand," I said. "And in answer to your question, yes, I'm now completely fine."

"Now tell me, how *is* your brother these days?" she asked with a funny sort of a smile.

"I wouldn't know," I replied with a funny sort of a smile back. "I haven't seen or heard from him in ages."

"Well, that's just fine," she said, "but promise you'd let me know if he ever comes a knocking again," and I was very happy to make that promise with every fiber of my being.

"Good," she said a little sadly, "because I just couldn't bear to lose a second man in my life."

"I'll drink to that," I agreed, and we clinked glasses.

▪ ▪ ▪

Some years before that evening on the Seine, I had been on a holiday to New York. While I was there, I was taken by a friend to the Yankee Stadium to watch a ball game. To the great distress of the home crowd, I witnessed the boys in the pin-striped pajamas get whacked by the visiting Red Sox.

It was a memorable evening, but for something that happened off the field rather than for anything that happened on it. At the end of the sixth innings, the large scoreboard blanked itself out all the usual and, to me, completely incomprehensible baseball statistics, and lit up with the simple message, "Shona, will you marry me?"

To my immense surprise and delight, the fellow sitting directly in front of me got out of his seat, turned to the girl sitting next to him, knelt on the concrete step, and presented her with an open jewelry box containing a large diamond ring. In between floods of tears, she said yes, of course, and her answer was relayed to the big screen, where it was greeted with a great cheer by fifty thousand people.

I had been mightily impressed. I realized that I might never get Helen to a baseball game, but since I had come to Paris with a particular purpose in mind, I was determined to do the best that I could under the circumstances. As a result, between the entree and the main course, and to the enthusiastic applause of our fellow diners, I did the knee-and-box thing by our table.

After she'd repaired her mascara, Helen, just like the girl at the Yankee stadium, then said yes to yet further applause. The only downside to the whole episode being that, in the excitement of the moment, Helen completely lost her appetite and wasn't able to eat so much of an atom of the exquisitely expensive meal that was put in front of her just a few moments later.

"You should have proposed after we'd finished eating," she said as she dabbed her face.

"No way," I replied. "I've already waited far too long."

After I finished eating both of our meals, Helen and I went up to the open-air top deck. Paris looked stunning. The Eiffel Tower was all lit up, and as we stood there, the whole city put on a spectacular fireworks display.

"They've really done all this just for us?" I asked in awe and was quite disappointed when I found out that it was also Bastille Day.

When the fireworks were over, Helen went down to powder her nose. On my own, I looked up at the moon above and felt like singing to a small guitar. "Thank you, thank you," I said, looking up at the night sky with my arms wide open. "Thank you to whatever it is that sticks everything together."

"What on earth are you doing?" Helen said when she came back and caught me in the act.

"Saying thank you," I said.

"What for?" she asked.

"For you," I replied simply, and she snuggled up against me.

"You realize this means I'll want you to come back to Australia with me," I said as we walked home along cobbled streets.

"Of course," she replied and tightened her arm around mine.

"But what about the girls?" I asked.

"I'm hoping you'll agree for them to come back and live with us too," Helen replied, glancing up at me, and I told her that would be just fine.

Then I had a thought. "But what about your brother?" I asked.

"I'll speak to him tomorrow," Helen replied. "I actually think he'll be delighted. It'll allow him to get on with both his research and his personal life uninterrupted."

"And the girls?" I persisted.

"I'm sure they'll love the idea," she reassured me. "Anyway, my brother is always visiting Australia on university business. They'll probably see at least as much of him living there as they do here."

When we got back to the apartment, we stood on the steps and kissed for a while in the cool night air.

"Helen," I eventually said when she got out her keys to open the door. "Before we go in, there is something I want to say. Something that I have to share with you."

"And what's that?" she looked up and asked a little apprehensively. "Having come all this way to see you, and in the hope that you *now* are ready," I continued, "it is not my intention to sleep in the guest room tonight."

"Oh," she said quietly, and she blushed as she unlocked the door to let us in.

22

MURRAY

I am sitting on the top deck of a riverboat, watching the bush slide slowly by on either side while Nel sleeps in the sun on the deck beside me. Pelicans swim out of our way as we surge forward, swallows hunt for insects in front of the bows, and a pair of eagles circles the thermals overhead. The sky is an unblemished dome of blue, and the river is a perfect mirror of pale opalescent brown. The only breeze is caused by the movement of the boat, and the only noise is the rhythmic throbbing of the engine.

The girls are steering and have been for the last hour or so. They must be doing it well, for I haven't heard any squabbling, and so far at least, we haven't hit anything. I am not sure where Helen is, probably curled up with a crossword or having a bit of a snooze.

It has been a wonderful honeymoon. There has been plenty of time for relaxation, and with none of the usual tugs and intrusions of everyday life.

"It must be past six somewhere in the world," I say to myself as I pour myself a glass of wine and settle deeper into the seat under the awning.

■ ■ ■

Just one week before, the day had dawned in an unpromising way. It had been quite overcast, and a cold wind had been blowing from the southeast.

I had looked anxiously at the sky as I scurried around, performing the many chores I still had to do to get the garden ready. I needn't have worried, however, for by midmorning the clouds had all vanished. By lunchtime, the winds that had blown the clouds away had also disappeared, and by afternoon, when things were scheduled to get underway, it was one of those warm, still spring days that Victoria does so well.

The crowd had started to assemble much earlier than I had expected, and even before the guest of honor arrived, they had dug deeply into the stocks of champagne and peaches. By the time that Helen eventually came up the driveway in the Bentley we had borrowed from a friend, everyone was well oiled.

Helen's yes on the boat on the Seine had sparked an amazing flurry of activity on my part. I was keen to make everything happen quickly so that there was to be no possibility of her slipping through my fingers again.

Even before leaving Paris, we decided on the garden at Woongarra for the ceremony. On my return, I was therefore plunged into a world of marquees, portaloos, refrigerated trailers, mobile kitchens, dance floors, and trying to work out how best to get the piano outside and still in tune. *How* we got married seemed to be an even more complex process than that of finding one another in the first place.

In the event, however, everything went off just perfectly. On the edge of the lake near the house and in front of all our friends, Helen and I pledged ourselves to one another for the rest of our lives, and the girls acted as bridesmaids.

Father Padraig looked after the ceremony, Pamela and Carmen looked after the food, Hugo and Reggy fussed over our mothers, Mung shook my hand several times, and Phill looked after the drinks. At least, at the beginning he did, but having adopted a "one for you and one for me" policy right from the start, he lost the ability to perform his duties midway through the afternoon and spent the rest of the time sitting and chatting with the guests while I ran around doing the honors.

Usually, Phill is the darling of any party, but this time he was pushed into second place. Looking magnificent in her bandana and black dreadlocks, Nel not only won everyone's hearts, but also cleaned up after them all as well.

The wedding presents were meant to be "something for the cellar or something for the garden." My friends all gave bottles while Helen's friends all gave trees. The presents were laid out on Gazza's table. It was the presents which we had imagined would be "ooed" and "aahed" over, but it was the table which was admired by all.

"We heard you made that," people said admiringly as they pointed at the table.

"Well, sort of," I replied quietly while looking round to make sure that Gazza wasn't within earshot.

And then Helen and I wandered round the garden thanking everyone for coming. There was Ruby, there was Heather and Rob and Meaghan, there was Ewa and Andre, there was Nigel and Riz, there was Andrew, there was Mario and Constanza, there was Rita, and there were many, many more.

Helen had loved her present of the piano. I had started out by thinking that, with a bit of practice, it wouldn't take me long to give Duke Ellington a nudge, but I never got beyond *Three Blind Mice*. I worked hard enough at it, but maybe I started too late or my fingers are wired-up back to front. Either way, I eventually came to realize that the Duke had no need to look over his shoulder as far as I was concerned, and simply tied it up with a large white satin bow for the big day. Unlike me, Helen brings out the best that Enzo's and Umberto's piano has to offer. She fills the house with Mozart and his friends. Not quite on a daily basis, but pretty much close to.

Late in the afternoon, Helen and I came across Darryl and Rosemary sitting quietly under the shade of a tree.

"Well, you've found your peace now, Paul," Rosemary said, and I couldn't but agree with her.

Eventually, Helen and I decided that we'd shaken enough hands and been hugged and kissed enough, and that it was time for everyone to look after themselves. Hand in hand, and with the girls in tow, we wandered for the last time among the guests and bid everyone farewell. When we had completed our adieus, I stood for a moment, looking back at the crowd still busily chatting on the lawn.

"Something missing?" asked Helen.

"Someone," I said with a sigh. "I would have liked Mark to be here today," I added.

"But then again," Helen said gently with that breathtaking intuition of hers, "maybe he *was* here and you just didn't notice him."

▪ ▪ ▪

The riverboat rounds a bend, and with the change of direction, a pleasant breeze cools my cheek. As the boat settles into the new straight, I shift my seat to stay in the shade, sip my drink, and smile at all that has happened.

Since leaving England, it has certainly been a journey of twists and turns. It has never been dull, and I have met many wonderful people along the way.

For over a quarter of a century, I have been privileged to serve a small rural community in a hidden away place on the other side of the globe. Though close to Melbourne, it is as if it has been locked in a time warp, away from the ebb and flow of history and preserved as a diorama of an old- fashioned, gentler, more caring world.

There has been plenty of laughter, and there has certainly also been a few tears. I have loved, almost, every bit of it. I hope that there is plenty more to come, and I wouldn't have missed any of it for quids.

And now, with the sun low on the horizon, I can see that the girls have us headed for a mooring spot on the bank. I get up, stretch, and nudge the dog awake, for we had better go down and give a hand.

As we near the bank, I hear shouts from a nearby houseboat and, looking across, realize that they had intended using the same mooring spot that we have beaten them to.

"Should we move over and let them in?" Lucy asks.

"Don't be silly," I reply, "first come, first served."

"But mightn't they be cross with us?" Imogen chips in.

"They might be," I say, "but just remember, girls—" I start to add, but I didn't get any further.

"What other people think of us is none of our business," they cut in and chanted with a sigh, and then jumped ashore and tied the boat up for the night.

www.ingramcontent.com/pod-product-compliance
Ingram Content Group UK Ltd.
Pitfield, Milton Keynes, MK11 3LW, UK
UKHW020425250726
13967UKWH00007B/2820